Endorsements from Medical Professionals

Sheryl Ellinwood boldly covers two crucial healthcare topics—personal responsibility and prevention. These topics are under the rubric of breast cancer, but the book also provides guidance for any disease state, for the maintenance of health in general, and for the prevention of disease. As such, *Empowered* is a must-read!

    PETER BOELENS, MD, MPH

An excellent resource for women and their physicians. A practical, well-written discussion of important research that every woman should be made aware of ! I recommend it highly.

    CELESTE HUGHES, N.D., H.H.P

    DOCTOR OF NATUROPATHY

    HOLISTIC HEALTHCARE PRACTITIONER

I wholeheartedly endorse *Empowered* as a thorough and well-written book. It includes a wealth of information on how to prevent breast cancer, including ways to strengthen the immune system—a strengthening that would, of course, prevent more than just breast cancer. The book's advice to guide women with breast cancer through treatment, with an appropriate emphasis on getting a second opinion, is excellent.

    CHARLES SCHAFER MD, DABS

    AUTHOR OF *HEALTH AND HUMOR*

Empowered

A Woman-to-Woman Guide
to Preventing and Surviving Breast Cancer

By Sheryl Ellinwood

Published and printed in the United States of America by The Write Place. For more information, please contact:

The Write Place
599 228th Place
Pella, Iowa 50219
www.thewriteplace.biz

ISBN: 978-0-9800084-7-0

Cover and interior art: Jan Gipple, www.jangipple.com
Interior design by Alexis Thomas, The Write Place

Copies of this book may be ordered at www.pinkempower.com.
They may also be mail ordered from ellinwood studios at a cost of $12.00 each.

Send check or money order to:
ellinwood studios, inc.
PO Box 197
Pella, IA 50219

For one to two books, add $3.00 shipping fee. For three or more books sent to the same address, shipping is free.

Acknowledgements

I never thought I would write a book. But I never thought I would get breast cancer either. Both have been learning experiences that required the help and support of others. I am grateful for all the love and support I received from family and friends, and even from business associates, after learning of my breast cancer diagnosis. Their well-wishes meant a great deal to me.

This book would not be in its present form if it weren't for the keen eye of my editor Carol Van Klompenburg. She not only made all the beneficial suggestions a great editor should make; she also edited the book through the lens of a breast cancer survivor—being one herself. Carol's staff at The Write Place helped with the fine-tuning of the text and greatly enhanced the cover design. Without the contributions of Donna Biddle and Alexis Thomas, this book would have suffered.

I am also grateful for the discerning eye of Alice Shives, my friend and proofreader who caught anything the rest of us missed. Special thanks goes to my friend and artist, Jan Gipple, for her work creating the cover design and allowing the use of her artwork on the cover and throughout the book. I also thank her for all the wonderful lunches she made whenever we had a "book meeting." I am appreciative of the time Debbie Markham spent working late at night to hone the cover text and design.

I am indebted to all the women who answered my breast cancer survey. They did not know me and still trusted me with their very personal information.

I am grateful to the doctors I met who answered my questions, considered the studies I brought to their attention, and took the time to hear me. I learned from them, and I hope they learned from me. I am especially indebted to all of the physicians and scientists I cite in this book, because this book could not have been written without their research.

Most of all I have to thank my husband, Jerome Keller, who supports me in whatever I do and lets me keep every stray cat that comes my way.

Disclaimer

This book is based on the author's personal experience and research. Neither the author nor the publisher is a health care provider. This book was written for informational and educational purposes only and not intended to be used as medical advice.

The author and publisher make no representation or warranties of any kind with respect to this book and its contents. The author and publisher do not represent or warrant that the information accessible through this book is accurate, complete, or current.

Neither the author nor publisher, nor any contributors or other authors cited will be liable for any damages arising from the use of this book. This is a comprehensive limitation of liability and applies to damages of any kind.

Statements made about products and services have not been evaluated by the Food and Drug Administration. They are not intended to diagnose, treat, cure, or prevent any disease or condition. This book is not intended as a substitute for consultation with a licensed health care practitioner. Before you start any health care program or lifestyle changes, you should consult with a health care practitioner to ensure that you are in good health and that examples contained in this book will not hurt you.

The reader's use of this book implies acceptance of this disclaimer.

Contents

Introduction 8

1. The Crucial First Step: Deciding to Ask Questions 11

2. Doing Your Own Research: Why and How 17

3. Cancer Cells: A Breakdown of Defense 29

4. Prevention: Your Breasts Are What You Eat 35

5. Prevention: Supplements and Lifestyle 55

6. Hormones: The Elephant in the Room 69

7. Who Controls Your Cancer Treatment? 83

8. Help Your Doctor Heal You 91

9. Chemotherapy: A Near-Death Experience 99

10. Radiation: The Nuclear War on Cancer 111

11. Mastectomy: The Removal of Fear 119

12. Breast Cancer Prevention Action Plan 127

13. Postscript 131

Meet the Author 135

Index 136

Introduction

Like most women, when I learned I had breast cancer I was suddenly confronted with test results, pathology reports, and a host of terms whose meaning and significance I didn't understand. My doctors spoke a foreign language. And although I was befuddled, I was expected to make decisions about treatments with serious health consequences that would affect me for the rest of my life.

Hearing that I had breast cancer was like suddenly being dropped into a foreign land where I didn't understand the customs or speak the language. When I have traveled to foreign countries, I have learned not to just shake my head in agreement when I don't understand what I am being asked or told, at least not if I don't want to end up in an uncomfortable or dangerous situation. Before I travel, I research the history of the country, its religious beliefs and customs, its political structure, tourist warnings, and current events. I also learn enough of its language for basic communication. I have traveled to dangerous countries like South Africa, but because of my research, I have always returned home safely.

When I found myself in the foreign country of breast cancer, I knew I needed to do research. I had to learn the language, the history and politics, and gain an awareness of the hidden dangers, along with current treatments and studies—if I wanted to return home safely.

To prepare for travel, I found books by writers who have lived in and experienced a country and compiled all that research in a handy guidebook. But I could find no such book for the land of breast cancer. I found plenty of information on individual breast cancer topics, but no guidebook that put all the facts together in an accessible format. I realized I needed to make one for myself.

As I was learning about breast cancer, I also learned I was not alone. I was amazed that almost every woman I talked with either had had breast cancer or knew someone who had. When I started talking to breast cancer survivors, I found that many of them didn't understand their disease. They were intelligent women, but because much information about breast cancer is highly technical, they had simply trusted their doctors to understand their disease and treat it. They didn't do much in-depth research on their own. Many simply turned to either the National Cancer Institute or the American Cancer Society for information, unaware of the financial ties these organizations have to the companies that make the drugs that treat cancer as well as the toxic chemicals that actually cause cancer. They also were not aware of proven ways to prevent breast cancer occurrence or recurrence.

After thoroughly researching these topics because of my own breast cancer, I realized that many women could use the information I had discovered, and *Empowered: A Woman-to-Woman Guide to Preventing and Surviving Breast Cancer* was born.

In these pages, I do not diagnose your disease or prescribe treatments. I take some very complicated information on breast cancer treatment and prevention and make it more understandable. I provide information that you are not likely to obtain from your doctors or from the major cancer organizations.

I offer crucial basic information and then show you how to conduct additional research on your own, directing you to the resources to use as a starting point. Each page has a column that lists resources for further research and also provides space for you to write notes. For easier access to the Web sites listed, links to all of these URLs are posted at www.pinkempower.com.

My goal for *Empowered* is to help women with cancer diagnoses to make wise treatment decisions, and to help women make decisions that will prevent the disease from recurring, or from occurring for the first time.

I wrote this book for women who wonder deep down whether they should question the current standard of care for breast cancer. I wrote this book for women who want to research prevention choices and treatment options.

If you are one of them, this book is for you.

Sheryl Ellinwood

September 2009

There's nothing that will lead to better medical care than a knowledgeable patient.

DR. C. EVERETT KOOP, FORMER SURGEON GENERAL

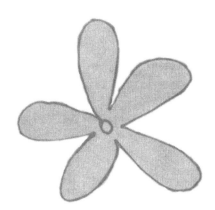

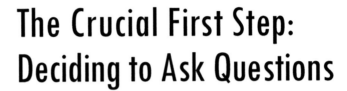

The Crucial First Step: Deciding to Ask Questions

Yes, I am a breast cancer survivor, but I'm not writing a tale about my disease. I'm sharing what I learned as I struggled to make good decisions about treatment. And I'm challenging women to do their own learning about prevention and treatment of breast cancer. As women, we can empower ourselves with knowledge, and acquiring that knowledge requires work. It requires suspending our belief that doctors always know best.

I believe that acquiring that knowledge and suspending that belief saved my life.

Two days before my bilateral mastectomy, my doctor asked me if I was "comfortable" with my decision to have both breasts removed. Truth be told, I would have rather buried my head in the sand and done nothing, hoping that my healthy eating, excellent physical health, and positive attitude would rid my body of these misbehaving cells.

But I answered that, yes—I was comfortable with my decision to have a mastectomy because I knew what I was doing. Most importantly—after months of research on the Internet, reading stacks of books, deciphering medical studies and pathology reports, challenging my doctors, and following my own intuition and intelligence—I knew why I was doing it. I knew a double

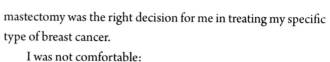

mastectomy was the right decision for me in treating my specific type of breast cancer.

I was not comfortable:

- Knowing that if symptoms elsewhere in my body had been properly treated years earlier, I might not have developed breast cancer.
- That my doctors did not know about studies documenting ways to prevent breast cancer when it is not genetic—and 90 percent of all breast cancer is not genetic.
- With the omission of information about the huge risks associated with the treatments I had been offered.
- With the doctors who thought I should not question them.
- That I had needed to do the research I had thought my doctors would do.

Most of all, I was not comfortable with the knowledge that, like me, women in the United States diagnosed with breast cancer will eventually confront the "standard of care" practiced in this country.

That standard of care typically includes some of the following:

- Biopsy and lumpectomy
- Radiation
- Tamoxifen—if the cancer is hormone receptive
- Chemotherapy
- Mastectomy
- Subsequent annual mammogram

This standard of care does seem to be a plan. And when diagnosed with breast cancer, a woman wants a plan. She wants action, and she wants to be rid of the cancer. She trusts that her doctors know what they are doing, are aware of all the alternatives, are familiar with all the current studies and information, and that they are investing time reviewing her specific case.

That's their job. Who would question them? Who would question the established system of cancer treatment? If you want to prevent breast cancer or make sure you have the best treatment for your specific type of breast cancer, the answer to these questions should be: You!

I did question. Eventually, I became an informed patient who understood the risks and benefits of each recommended procedure and treatment before giving my consent. I investigated other, less toxic treatments and considered them. I learned to prepare for each doctor's visit with a list of questions or concerns. I learned to trust my instinct when something just didn't feel right. And I learned that it is both unfair and unwise to place the entire burden for our medical care on our doctors.

As I studied, I began to understand the financial link between pharmaceutical companies, The National Cancer Institute, The American Cancer Society, the institutions that educate doctors, and the Food and Drug Administration (FDA)—a link that makes it unlikely women receive the most appropriate treatment. I discovered why valuable information that can prevent breast cancer or treat it in a non-toxic way does not reach women or their doctors.

Once I understood how doctors are trained, and how they think, I was not afraid to question them and to help them heal me, not simply treat me. Seeing the whole picture equipped me to work with my doctors to make the best decisions regarding my treatment.

I want to share the results of my research with other women. I also want to teach them how to research for themselves both how to prevent breast cancer and how to avoid getting a one-size-fits-all treatment that may actually cause their breast cancer to recur.

The United States has the highest rate of breast cancer in the world. One out of every seven women in this country will be diagnosed with breast cancer, and that rate is climbing. We are no closer to a cure for breast cancer than we were twenty years ago. Women are being subjected to harmful treatments that offer no long-term survival benefits. It's time for change. It's time for women to:

- Challenge the current treatment methods.
- Demand that more funding be directed towards prevention.
- Make changes in our lifestyles that will prevent breast cancer. (Women with unhealthy lifestyles are twice as likely to develop cancer.)
- Take the time to educate ourselves about treatment and prevention.
- Work in partnership with our doctors to decide the best course of treatment for each of us as individual women, not as statistics.

For a long and fascinating history of one breast cancer treatment, read "Revisiting Accepted Wisdom in The Management of Breast Cancer" by Harriet Beinfield, LAC, and Malcolm S. Beinfield, MD, FACS, printed in *Alternative Therapies*, September 1997, vol. 3, no. 5. Online, it can be found at: www.breastcancerchoices.org under "Resources."

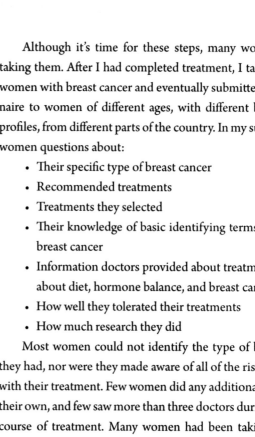

Although it's time for these steps, many women are not taking them. After I had completed treatment, I talked to many women with breast cancer and eventually submitted a questionnaire to women of different ages, with different breast cancer profiles, from different parts of the country. In my survey, I asked women questions about:

- Their specific type of breast cancer
- Recommended treatments
- Treatments they selected
- Their knowledge of basic identifying terms for types of breast cancer
- Information doctors provided about treatment risks and about diet, hormone balance, and breast cancer
- How well they tolerated their treatments
- How much research they did

Most women could not identify the type of breast cancer they had, nor were they made aware of all of the risks associated with their treatment. Few women did any additional research on their own, and few saw more than three doctors during the entire course of treatment. Many women had been taking synthetic hormones (hormone replacement therapy) prior to their breast cancer diagnoses, and only one woman's doctor explained the connection between hormones, hormone imbalance and breast cancer, even though the majority of women surveyed actually had symptoms of a hormonal imbalance prior to their breast cancer diagnoses. Only one woman's doctor ever talked to her about her diet in regards to her breast cancer. Almost half of the women surveyed were put on Tamoxifen.

What perplexes me about these results is that, with one exception, all twenty women I surveyed felt they were fully informed before making their decisions regarding treatment. Yet the inability of almost every one of them to answer even basic questions regarding their breast cancer diagnoses, pathology, or treatment risks indicates that they had not received complete or adequate information. They had a false sense of security. Based on the survey answers, what made these women feel they were fully informed was simply the trust they had that their doctors had told them everything they needed to know.

I saw clearly that, for women to begin to manage their own health, especially when faced with a breast cancer diagnosis, a huge first step is to realize that the nearly total reliance they place on their doctors as their sole source of information is unwise.

When it comes to any complex subject, and breast cancer is definitely complex, reliance on any single source of information can be dangerous. On a complex subject such as breast cancer, new discoveries are continually made, treatment recommendations reexamined, and new study results are published. Breast cancer treatment today is radically different from twenty years ago. Twenty years from now, today's treatments will be seen as radical and ineffective. The practice of medicine has a long history of proving that prior methods of treatment were ineffective—or even harmful. Women don't need to distrust all doctors, but they do need to realize that medical information is not absolute. It is a constantly changing and evolving field. Because of that change, it is always in your best interest to do your own research.

Once you venture out of the comfort zone of simply relying on your doctor and start doing your own research, your eyes will be opened to the vast amount of new information on breast cancer prevention and treatment options. You will find it helpful and empowering, and it will allow you to make a truly informed decision about your own breast cancer prevention and treatment.

And, just as you should not rely on your doctor as a sole source of information, you should not rely solely on me. Part of being an informed patient is to go beyond this book directly to the sources I cite and Google these terms yourself. I invite you to scrutinize and question the information I'm offering, and I ask you also to scrutinize the information your doctors provide and to ask them questions.

Questions may save your life. I believe they saved mine.

Are you still hesitant to question your doctor? You may want to read *The 10 Best Questions for Surviving Breast Cancer* by Dede Bonner, PhD.

Reason and free inquiry are the only effective agents against errors.

THOMAS JEFFERSON

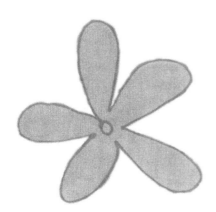

Doing Your Own Research: Why and How

In their research paper, "Revisiting Accepted Wisdom in the Management of Breast Cancer," Harriet Beinfield, LAC, and Malcolm S. Beinfield, MD, FACS, wrote, "Patients have the right of treatment choice, but most women are so poorly informed that they cannot choose wisely." Doing your own research is the key both to getting the best—the most appropriate, least damaging—treatment possible and to avoiding a breast cancer diagnosis in the first place.

The United States has the highest breast cancer occurrence rate in the world. It also has one of the highest death rates from breast cancer. This may be an indication that the best treatment might not be found in standard medical care. A physician might not make the best recommendation for your treatment. On average, a physician takes fifteen minutes to analyze your individual pathology in order to make a treatment recommendation. Often, it is during your appointment that a doctor reviews your pathology reports for the first time. Physicians say each cancer is unique, but they don't treat it uniquely. They want to select appropriate treatment, but the system doesn't allot time for you as an individual. Your doctor must try to lump you and your cancer into a certain "profile," whether or not you fit exactly. In fact, specific, documented modes of thinking actually prevent

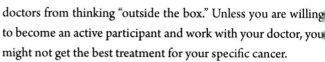

doctors from thinking "outside the box." Unless you are willing to become an active participant and work with your doctor, you might not get the best treatment for your specific cancer.

Current standard-of-care treatments for breast cancer are toxic (drugs, chemotherapy, radiation) or invasive (mastectomy). All have undesirable side effects and life-changing consequences. And they are not reversible. So it is important to know all the risks, benefits, side effects, and alternative treatments in order to make the right decision for yourself. Your doctor is not likely to tell you as much as you can learn through your own research. Many doctors are not even aware of the alternative, less damaging but equally effective treatments. Or, physicians may know about them and how effective they are, but are afraid of a lawsuit if they don't give you "standard care."

Do doctors resent proactive patients? Although some may, most do not. I asked my doctors if my questions bothered them. Most said that my questions made them consider new angles and information, which affected their ultimate treatment recommendations.

Many women with a breast cancer diagnosis conclude they don't have the time to spend doing research because they have to make a quick decision. However, unless you have an extremely aggressive cancer, you have at least a month, and often longer, to take the time to do the research to make a right decision, not just a quick one.

USE GOOGLE'S SEARCH ENGINE

The Internet is a superb research tool. Of course, you cannot believe everything you read there, and you are wise to distrust any site that is selling something. Information on any site should be verified by several other sites. Specific medical Web sites from the leading cancer hospitals such as Johns Hopkins, Memorial Sloan-Kettering, and Mayo Clinic are important, but do not limit your search to those sites. Search beyond the borders of the United States. European countries, which are ahead of the United States in cancer treatment, can provide very valuable data.

Begin your Internet research with selective Google searches. Researching is like a tree: you start with the trunk (your diagnosis) and then branch out. Each search will turn up information that will create another area for research. If you come across words you need defined, Google those words, too.

My initial diagnosis was DCIS (ductal carcinoma in situ). So, I started Google research with the following searches:

- What is DCIS?
- Is DCIS cancer?
- How is DCIS treated?
- Causes of DCIS
- Studies done on treatments for DCIS
- Prognosis for DCIS
- How is DCIS treated in Europe?
- Alternative treatments for DCIS
- Does radiation cure DCIS?
- Can radiation therapy cause cancer?

Each of those searches provided enough information to generate another search and so on.

BOOK SEARCHES

You can also use Amazon.com in the same way you use Google. You can search for books on any topic you wish. As your Internet research expands, you may find that you are interested in delving deeper into a certain topic. Books can provide this in-depth information on topics of special relevance to your cancer research. Be sure to check copyright and publication dates; older books will not have the most current discoveries.

STUDY YOUR PATHOLOGY REPORTS

To understand your specific breast cancer, you need to understand your pathology reports, so ask your doctor for a copy of each one.

Do not expect your doctor to fully explain this report to you. At first its words and sentences will be incomprehensible, but after you Google each word or phrase, you will eventually be able to decipher it.

Your pathology report may include the following terms:

- ER2: estrogen receptors, + or -
- PR2: progesterone receptors, + or -
- HER-2/neu: a specific growth protein receptor, + or -

- Triple Negative: negative for the three receptors above
- Nuclear Grade: a specific rating system where a higher rating indicates a more aggressive cancer
- Comedo Necrosis: a buildup of dead cancer cells
- DCIS: Ductal carcinoma in situ, means pre-cancerous cells contained within the milk ducts
- Invasive Cancer: cancer cells that have spread beyond the milk ducts into breast tissue
- Margins: the area of cancer-free tissue surrounding the original lump or tumor. You want 10 mm or more of clear margin. Think of your breast cancer as an egg; the yolk is the tumor and the egg white surrounding it is the margin.

You can Google each term above for more complete information.

As you become more familiar with the language of pathology reports, you will better understand each subsequent report. You may even notice that information is missing and request it. Following my lumpectomy for a .6 cm (6 mm) tumor determined to be DCIS, pathologists found a .5 cm (5 mm) invasive cancer tumor that had not shown up on a mammogram, ultrasound, or MRI. The medical system does not automatically cover all bases—the pathology report did not indicate hormone receptor status for this invasive tumor, crucial information for treatment. I asked my doctor to request that profile from the pathology laboratory. Had I not taught myself how to read the basics of the pathology reports, I would not have known enough to request that crucial information.

MEDICAL STUDIES

In your Internet searches you will come across many medical studies that have been published in leading medical journals such as the *Journal of the American Medical Association* (JAMA), *The American Journal of Surgery, New England Journal of Medicine (Journal Watch), American Society of Clinical Oncology, The Lancet,* and the *Annals of Surgical Oncology.* Do not skip these studies simply because they are hard to understand. Even though they are usually lengthy and chock full of medical jargon, they can be like gold. These studies provide evidence that a certain treatment works or does not work. You can speed your process by scrolling to the conclusion or summary at the end of the study and reading that first. It is usually a single paragraph or two that summarizes the study results. This paragraph tells you whether that particular study contains information you need. If it does, print it and invest time in deciphering it.

Most doctors are familiar with only several of the large studies done on breast cancer. These are the NSABP (National Surgical Adjuvant Breast Project) studies. Often, subsequent studies have been done that challenge the results, offer better and less toxic treatments, or even show that a prior treatment thought to work actually does not. For example, a new study done by the National Cancer Institute now shows that after being used for twelve years, Taxol, a widely used chemotherapy drug for breast cancer that also goes by several other names, is not effective for women with HER2-negative breast cancer.

You should also be aware of the difference between *in vitro* and *in vivo* studies. In vitro studies are studies done in petri dishes or test tubes in a lab, usually on cancer cells. While these studies may be promising, they don't really prove anything because they have not been tested in rats or humans. Something that works in the lab may not actually work in a more complex environment like a human body. Therefore, search for studies that have been done on rats (their breast physiology is the closest to the human body—who knew?) or even better yet, studies done on humans. These are called *in vivo* studies.

When it comes to studies, size matters. The larger the study (the more women involved) the better. Also, look for the word randomized in the study. If the study was randomized, in the group of women studied, half were given a placebo (a placebo is an empty pill—meaning they were given no treatment at all even though they thought they were) and the other half were given the drug or treatment being studied. Who gets the drug and who gets the placebo is essentially determined by a flip of a coin. This way there is no bias in who gets the treatment and who does not, so the results usually aren't skewed by other factors. Most often the first paragraph of the study will indicate the size of the study, if this was a study done in humans, and if it was randomized (also called double-blind).

Do not, however, totally dismiss any study that was not randomized. There are some very good studies done by some leading breast cancer doctors who have looked at the real life effects of treatments on women with breast cancer over the course of their medical practices and have discovered and documented some very important findings. Personally, I find those studies to be of great significance.

Beware of studies funded by the drug companies themselves, or just as bad, but harder to detect, studies done by physicians who are on the payroll or boards of those pharmaceutical companies. Those studies are most likely rigged to favor the drug being studied. It is easy to rig a study, and the most often utilized technique is that of giving only the healthiest women the drug being studied because if you are healthier, you have a much higher chance of surviving any negative side effects and a higher chance of a better overall outcome altogether. If a Google search results in any information with a drug company name attached to it, I pay little attention to that information. If that information or study is valid, it will show up elsewhere from less biased sources.

Many women rely on The American Cancer Society (ACS) or the National Cancer Institute (NCI) for all of their research and consider themselves to be fully informed. While these organizations do provide useful information and I do suggest that you use them as resources, I warn against relying on their information too heavily. Both of these organizations are headed by representatives of the large pharmaceutical industry, have worked to block efforts geared towards prevention, and actually lobby in favor of companies that produce the toxic chemicals linked to causing breast cancer. The information provided by these organizations may paint treatments by drug companies such as chemotherapy and radiation in a more favorable light than studies actually prove.

YOUR DOCTOR'S REACTION

Be warned, though, that even if you present your doctor with the most up-to-date, large, randomized human study done by a recognized cancer institution, he or she will most likely try to dismiss it. Doctors do this by reciting medical jargon that they know you will not understand, so you then think, "OK, they must be familiar with this study and know something more about it than I do." You just may be wrong to think that. Just four out of the eight doctors I saw were willing to actually read and consider the studies I showed them. Three of those doctors then took the information in those studies into account when we further discussed my treatment options.

Here's what happened with the fourth doctor. After my mastectomy, my oncologist recommended something called adjuvant chemotherapy. This means that just in case they missed a cancer cell or two during my mastectomy surgery, they wanted me to do a series of six chemotherapy treatments. Well, understanding that we all have defective, potential cancer cells in our bodies all the time and that a healthy immune system will destroy them, I argued that it simply made no sense to me to invade my entire body with toxic chemotherapy chemicals that would destroy my immune system and damage healthy cells only to possibly kill a cancer cell that may or may not be there! My oncologist listened to my argument, said I did have a valid point, but printed out the list of chemotherapy drugs he would recommend for me. To be fair to him, I told him I would research the information. My research revealed that one of the chemotherapy drugs he would have put me on was the same one listed in the report by the National Cancer Institute as not being effective for women with HER2-negative breast cancer. (If the NCI makes a statement *against* the use of a certain drug, I take that seriously.) I had HER2-negative breast cancer! I emailed that NCI report to my oncologist. His reply shocked me. He said it was "interesting," but wouldn't change what he recommended.

I really wondered, "What does it take for a doctor to change?" I may have found that answer in the book, *Anti Cancer: A New Way of Life* by Dr. David Servan-Schreiber. A cancer survivor himself, he asked that very same question, and here is his answer:

"In medical culture, changes in recommendations given to patients are allowable in only one case and one alone: when there has been a series of 'double-blind' studies demonstrating the effectiveness of a treatment in humans." What this says is that until there are a series of double-blind studies done—which will take years—showing that Taxol is not effective for women with

The report about Taxol being ineffective treatment for HER-2/neu negative breast cancer can be found at: www.healthcentral. com/breast-cancer/ c/6362/14847/ taxol-breast/. Click on the included links for additional information.

HER2-negative breast cancer, this toxic drug will continue to be prescribed for those women by most oncologists.

Add to that the fact that many doctors today are beholden to pharmaceutical companies in some way, whether they know it or not. The drug companies educate them both by funding medical schools and later by presenting them with biased company-funded "studies." They wine-and-dine them, and quite often pay bonuses for every drug or chemo treatment they prescribe. With that sort of influence, doctors have a vested financial interest in ignoring any information that could cause them to stop prescribing a drug or treatment from which they receive financial rewards. If you think this doesn't apply to your doctor, just glance around the office and waiting room. Do you see glossy brochures advertising certain drugs or office equipment such as clocks, prescription pads, calendars, etc. bearing drug company logos? This may seem insignificant, but it is evidence that your doctor is being marketed to by a drug sales representative, and just as in politics, money buys influence.

EPIDEMIOLOGY

First, let me define this term for you. According to the *Oxford Dictionary*, epidemiology is the "study of the incidence and distribution of diseases, and their control and prevention." Think of the root word "epidemic." The science of epidemiology is focused on identifying widespread disease patterns and occurrences (cancer is now nearly an epidemic), its causes and its prevention. Unlike the medical studies listed above, this is not done through large, randomized human trials. It is done by studying populations where the disease is most prevalent and attempting to find the reason why. In searching for the cause of the disease, all things are considered; no stone is left unturned. This is quite different from the limited, and very focused, method of the medical studies listed above. It is often the evidence of the cause of a disease, discovered by the epidemiological studies, that prompts these more focused medical studies. But these studies happen only in cases where the potential for a patented drug is seen.

One of the primary areas of epidemiology is studying how different diets contribute to disease. These studies now show a definite causal relationship between diet and cancer. By comparing the diets of populations throughout the world of those with the highest cancer rates to those with the lowest, a definite conclusion has been made that what you eat can either promote or prevent cancer. Here's the problem. Your doctors don't know this conclusion or have read about these epidemiological studies that have been reported in all the major science and medical journals, but they will not relay this information to their patients or incorporate it into their practices until the big "medical studies" Dr. Servan-Schreiber referred to above are done.

Where are all the big medical studies on how diet affects your risk of breast cancer? Other than a few isolated research centers, nowhere. Here's why. Medical studies on humans can cost anywhere from 500 million to a billion dollars. This cost can be justified if, at the end of the process, a patentable drug is likely to be proven effective. Sales of that drug will far exceed the cost of the study. Because food cannot be patented, there is little willingness to spend that kind of money on medical studies when there is no money to be made in the end.

Personally, I see a great deal of importance in epidemiological studies. It is much more enlightening to look back over long periods of time, while studying population patterns that allow for the natural variances in human beings, to identify causes of disease. Studies that are too narrow and focused often miss the forest for the trees. Consider how the source of a cholera outbreak in London in 1854 was discovered by Dr. John Snow. By conducting his own epidemiological study, looking at death records and interviewing the local residents, he identified the source of the disease as the water from the local pump. Once the pump handle was removed, there were no additional cholera deaths. This proved his theory that cholera was a waterborne, contagious disease, common knowledge today. His theory was not accepted until 1883, almost 30 years later. Today epidemiology is responsible for identifying and controlling all epidemics, such as aflatoxin poisoning, the flu, including the most recent H1N1 flu, as well as detecting and preventing adverse reactions to vaccinations. If it weren't for epidemiological discoveries, much of the human population would have been wiped out by

disease. It is a shame that doctors are trained only to consider the more narrowly focused studies.

CHAT ROOMS

While chat rooms can be a source of emotional support they usually do not provide helpful information about treatment or prevention. In a few chat rooms women discuss treatment options, but the information is usually sketchy. Chat rooms do show that women intuitively know there has to be a better way they just didn't know how to find it.

For me, the saddest part of visiting chat rooms was reading women's stories of receiving standard treatments, thinking they were cured, and then learning they had a recurrence. I wished they had discovered earlier the importance of educating themselves regarding prevention.

HOW MY RESEARCH MAY HAVE SAVED MY LIFE

I had discovered the importance of educating myself early in my course of treatment. After I discovered a small lump in my left breast, which had not shown up on the mammogram I had a few months earlier, the lump was removed and biopsied. The pathology report came back showing high grade ductal carcinoma in situ (DCIS), a very common diagnosis since the advent of mammography. My doctor sent me to an oncologist who wanted to schedule me for immediate radiation treatments. I was concerned about the lack of time this doctor had spent reviewing my pathology report. I had done my own research on my pathology. After asking him a few questions, I realized I knew more than he did about the contents of my pathology report. I told him I believed radiation would do more harm than good. He replied, "I'm sorry, but then I can't help you. Have a nice day."

I knew I needed to find a different doctor, so I called a well-known breast cancer center in Iowa. I told the woman at the appointment desk I might be considered a difficult patient because I ask a lot of questions and do my own research. I asked for an appointment with a doctor open to that. She replied, "All good doctors welcome patient questions and input," and so I made an appointment.

Ten days later I met with a helpful doctor who discussed my odd pathology report, which had been so unusual it was sent to Mayo Clinic for assessment. He also listened to my objections to radiation and evaluated my stack of current DCIS studies. We agreed that before radiation was even considered, I needed to have a lumpectomy to determine tumor margins (the area of tissue free of cancer cells surrounding the original tumor). The first oncologist should have recognized the need for a lumpectomy before suggesting radiation treatments.

After the lumpectomy was performed, the biopsy came back showing insufficiently clear margins (anything less than 10 mm clear in all directions is not adequate), one more area of high grade DCIS, and a small invasive cancer tumor that was not detected even by the MRI. If I had immediately undergone radiation treatments as the first oncologist wanted, my invasive cancer would not have been discovered. Then, because of the tissue damage caused by the radiation, the invasive tumor would have been harder to detect and may not have been discovered until it was large enough to have spread to my lymph nodes.

I am a living example of the value of personal research.

For statistics on breast cancer rates and survival rates in the US and throughout the world visit:

- www.worldwidebreast cancer.com (click on the map)
- www.cancer.org
- www.breastcancer.org

I for one believe that if you give people a thorough understanding of what confronts them and the basic causes that produce it, they'll create their own program, and when the people create a program, you get action.

MALCOLM X

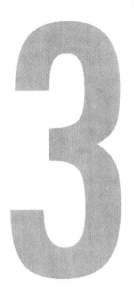

Cancer Cells:
A Breakdown of Defense

When we understand how breast cancer begins, we are empowered to make better choices for both treatment and prevention.

Put in very basic terms, all healthy cells in our bodies have a specific purpose. Cancer cells are unhealthy, damaged cells that have not matured into cells with a specific purpose. They are called undifferentiated. Healthy cells are called differentiated because each one has a different purpose in our body. Undifferentiated cells are confused about their purpose. They may be mildly confused and be called moderately differentiated, or extremely confused and be called poorly differentiated. If you have breast cancer, these terms should appear in your pathology report. (Poorly differentiated cancer cells are more aggressive.) Because these cells don't know what they are supposed to do, they simply keep growing and reproducing more damaged cells just like themselves which will eventually become a cancer tumor.

Healthy cells not only know what they are supposed to do, they know when they are supposed to die. This pre-programmed cell death is called apoptosis. Damaged cells that don't know their purpose, also don't know when to die. So they just keep growing and reproducing, some faster than others.

For a detailed medical explanation of how cancer begins, read *What Your Doctor May Not Tell You About Breast Cancer* by Dr. John Lee.

The good news is that our bodies have mechanisms to recognize these bad cells and target them for removal. Most of the time that system works beautifully. If it didn't, we'd all be filled with cancer. Sometimes our bodies miss a few bad cells or are tricked into not recognizing them, and they don't get destroyed. And cancer gets its start.

The three questions to ask about the start of cancer are:

- What causes these cells to be undifferentiated?
- What causes our bodies' seek-and-destroy mechanisms to fail?
- How can we prevent both of these things from happening?

Let's take those questions one at a time.

First, what causes cells to become undifferentiated? An undifferentiated, or damaged, cell is born when something alters the DNA (the control center) of that cell. Once the DNA has been altered, the cell malfunctions and reproduces more cells with that same damaged DNA. This damage can be caused by a carcinogen (cancer causing agent) such as:

- Toxins in our food and our environment
- Viruses
- Radiation

It can also be caused by:

- Hormonal imbalances
- Lack of specific nutrients in our diet
- Physical damage to the breast tissue

If your breast cancer is caused by a genetic mutation, you are born with the defective DNA. But only 10 percent of all breast cancer is genetic. All other breast cancers are caused by one or all of the above.

Second, what causes our bodies' natural seek-and-destroy mechanisms to fail? This mechanism, called our immune system, is a very complex system made up of different types of cells, mostly white blood cells. These include T cells, which are often referred to as "killer cells," macrophages, and neutrophils—but there are many others. These cells patrol the body looking for foreign substances or damaged cells. Once an invader or damaged cell is identified, it is destroyed—if our immune system is working properly. If our immune system has been weakened, invaders and damaged cells can go undetected and start an infection, disease, or cancer.

You are bound to encounter people who will cite others who tried to cure their cancer by using a natural approach using herbs or supplements and died. Without the specifics about their cancer, the product, and the dosage, such examples prove nothing. Yet some people use an example like this to dismiss all natural treatments. The same logic could be applied to any of the millions of women who died following standard treatment with radiation or chemotherapy. Women need facts about all their treatment options so that they can decide for themselves which treatment option to pursue.

For more information on the growth in alternative medicine, go to: http://health.usnews.com/articles/health/2008/01/09/embracing-alternative-care.html.

The wise man should consider that health is the greatest of human blessings. Let food be your medicine.

HIPPOCRATES

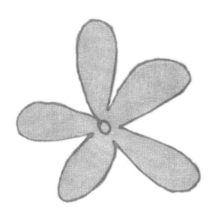

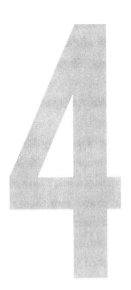

Prevention: Your Breasts Are What You Eat

Our bodies' natural defenses are the best mechanism for fighting cancer. Diet and lifestyle can weaken or boost our immune systems. Richard Beliveau, PhD, author of *Foods That Fight Cancer* and a specialist in cancer biology, concludes that the "principle difference between populations with the highest cancer rates and those with the lowest was their food."

In reference to what and how we eat in the United States (high sugar; bad fats; processed foods; toxin-laden meat, dairy, and produce) he states, "With all I've learned over these years of research, if I were asked to design a diet today that promoted the development of cancer to the maximum, I couldn't improve on our present diet!"

The American Institute for Cancer Research estimates that between 33 percent and 70 percent of all cancers are diet related. Many experts feel that rate is much higher. Although women are not to blame for developing breast cancer, they can lower their risk of occurrence or recurrence by identifying and changing the eating habits and lifestyles that may have caused the cancer to take hold.

Learning about the importance of diet and lifestyle is not for the purpose of finger-pointing or blaming; it's to empower yourself with the knowledge to prevent cancer. An imbalance in your

To learn more about how toxins accumulate and how this accumulation impacts our bodies, read *Experimental Man: What One Man's Body Says About His Future, Your Health, and Our Toxic World* by David Ewing Duncan. Duncan subjected his body to a multitude of tests for toxin content, and what he learned disturbed him.

In his book, *Foods That Fight Cancer*, Richard Beliveau, PhD, details his studies that determined which foods inhibited the growth of certain cancers. A complete list can be found in this book.

To learn more about environmental toxins, visit this Web site: www.ewg.org. For information about antioxidants, free radicals, and oxidation, visit:

www.glyconutrientsreference.com/.

weneedglyconutrients/toxinsandfreeradicals.php.

that have estrogen receptors, such as ER+ cells in breast tissue. But xenoestrogens are molecularly different from our natural estrogens, and they can have undesirable health consequences. This risk is similar to the difference and the dangers of synthetic hormones used in hormone replacement therapy. For example, the natural hormone progesterone protects against breast cancer, but the synthetic version called progestin causes breast cancer. Obviously, a woman who has ER+ (estrogen receptor positive) breast cancer should avoid xenoestrogens—both in food and in cosmetics.

SUGARS

If you can't eliminate refined sugars entirely from your diet, at least minimize your intake as much as possible.

Cancer cells love sugar! Otto Warburg, PhD, received the Nobel Prize in Medicine in 1931 for discovering that cancer cells have a very different metabolism than healthy cells. Cancer cells do not utilize oxygen in their metabolism as healthy cells do. Because sugars (glucose) do not need oxygen in order to be converted to energy, glucose is the "food of choice" for cancer cells. Cancer cells metabolize glucose at a rate four to five times higher than healthy cells.

While healthy cells also use sugars, they get much of their energy from fats and proteins, which require oxygen to metabolize. In fact, to locate metastasized cancer with a PET scan, a sugar solution with a radioactive tracer is injected into the body. Because the cancer cells metabolize sugar at a faster rate than healthy cells, they will take up the sugar-tracer solution quickly and show up on the scan.

A very recent discovery also shows that cancer cells produce a specific protein called Akt. This protein, which also requires glucose, may be what makes a cancer cell able to avoid apoptosis (the pre-programmed death in a healthy cell). Several studies have shown that in populations where women have a lower dietary sugar intake they have significantly lower rates of breast cancer. The above information may explain why.

Simple sugars are also harmful in other ways. When we eat refined or simple sugars, they go immediately from our digestive system into the bloodstream, quickly increasing blood sugar levels. Once sugars are in the bloodstream they are converted to glucose. Insulin, our blood-sugar-balancing hormone created in the pancreas, then rushes out into the bloodstream to escort the glucose into the cells. This big rush of insulin causes too much glucose to be moved out of the blood and that causes a sudden drop in blood sugar levels. That low blood sugar will cause many people to feel tired, dizzy, shaky, or moody. The most common reaction is to then eat something sugary to get blood sugar levels up again, and the cycle repeats.

This repeated cycle causes a condition called insulin resistance, where your insulin can no longer effectively get the glucose into your cells. People with insulin resistance have chronically high levels of both insulin and glucose in their blood; and both lead to a host of chronic health conditions including diabetes and breast cancer. Another result of insulin resistance is that more glucose gets stored as fat, especially around the midsection. Body fat produces estrogen, so increasing our body fat increases our estrogen production—and our risk of breast cancer.

Notice that above I talked about refined sugars or simple sugars (also called simple carbohydrates). Simple or refined sugars are different from complex sugars or carbohydrates in a very important way. Our bodies cannot be healthy without carbohydrates; along with fats and proteins they are what the body converts into energy. Complex carbohydrates have something that refined carbohydrates don't have: fiber. The fiber in complex carbohydrates helps the sugars to be absorbed slowly into your system preventing the rush of insulin caused by simple sugars. Eating complex carbohydrates can actually lower your insulin level. But, because complex carbohydrates are also sugars, it is not wise to eat a diet entirely of complex carbohydrates, especially if you want to prevent cancer. A healthy diet should include good fats, proteins, and complex carbohydrates.

Complex carbohydrates are found in whole foods such as fruits, vegetables, and whole grains. Simple carbohydrates are found in processed foods and include white sugars, brown sugars, corn syrup, molasses, maple syrup, honey, white rice, and anything made with white flour such as white pasta, white bread, cookies, cakes, pies, and most cereals. Fruit juices are simple carbohydrates because they have had all the fiber stripped away.

Here's a book to consider reading, especially for those diagnosed with breast cancer and undergoing radiation or chemotherapy treatments: *Natural Strategies for Cancer Patients*, by Dr. Russell L. Blaylock.

Here's another book I found worthwhile: *Anti-Cancer: A New Way of Life* by David Servan-Schreiber, MD.

Here's a helpful Web site on cancer and sugar: http://www.second-opinions.co.uk/cancer-5.html. Read the article, but also scroll down to the reference section and investigate some of the studies cited.

Be especially wary of whole wheat labels on breads and pastas. If it doesn't say 100 percent whole grain whole wheat, then it is most likely no better than white flour.

I also discovered firsthand that increased insulin can throw hormones out of balance. For me, that imbalance resulted in my developing uterine fibroid tumors eight years ago. I had always loved eating cakes, cookies, and ice cream. Because I had always been thin, I didn't think eating them mattered. By age forty, however, I had gained ten pounds in my butt, hip, and stomach area. I also developed uterine fibroids. At forty-six, my fibroid tumors had grown large enough to cause significant pain, and my doctor recommended a hysterectomy. I told her that I first wanted to research alternative treatments. A week later I stumbled across Suzanne Somers book, *Eat, Cheat, and Melt the Fat Away*. It caught my attention because the cover boasted of 100 delicious recipes, and I love to cook. However, the book opened to a chapter on hormone balance. I didn't think I had a hormone imbalance, but I read the chapter, and I'm glad I did. It taught me the relationship between my sugar intake and my fibroids. I learned that my fibroids were the result of a hormonal imbalance caused by insulin resistance.

I stopped eating refined sugars cold turkey! Within three months, I lost twelve pounds, and my fibroid tumors had shrunk to the point that they caused no pain. Eight years later, I still have not had that hysterectomy, and I am still symptom-free.

I regret that I did not notice at the time I was researching fibroids that there is also a link between hormonal levels and breast cancer. Because I had no family history of breast cancer and thought I had no risk factors, breast cancer wasn't on my radar. I certainly regret overlooking that information now! What I wish I had realized then was the need to get my hormone levels checked. You can never know for sure, but I certainly feel that if I had been properly diagnosed and treated for my hormonal imbalance, I may not have gotten breast cancer because a link between hormone imbalances and breast cancer has been established.

Besides refined sugar, it is wise to avoid foods ranked high on the glycemic index. In this index, the higher the number, the more that food increases your insulin level. With the exception of red wine (in moderation) and certain vegetables like carrots, beets, and squash, I try not to eat anything with a score higher than fifty.

It takes a strong will to say no to sugar, but once you stop eating refined sugars, in a short while your sugar cravings diminish and anything containing those refined sugars tastes much too sweet. You no longer have those blood sugar ups and downs caused by rapid fluctuations in your insulin, in which one minute you are fine and the next you are shaky and about to faint from hunger.

ARTIFICIAL SWEETENERS

It is impossible to give up eating everything sweet, however, so most people turn to artificial sweeteners. While all artificial sweeteners will prevent the insulin roller coaster ride, be wary of artificial sweeteners. Most are not found in nature, but are synthetic, chemical concoctions that can be harmful and contain toxins. If you want to prevent cancer, the last thing you want to do is put toxic chemicals into your body. I have found a few that are safe. Experiment with them to see which tastes best and works best for you.

Agave Nectar: This is juice from the agave plant (from which tequila is made) and is the consistency of honey and almost as sweet. It is not calorie-free, but is low on the glycemic index, so it won't spike your insulin. It can be used in baking, but because it is a liquid, you will have to cut the liquid in the recipe by one-third. Also use 25 percent less agave nectar than the sugar called for. Agave nectar can be found in health food stores, some upscale grocery stores, and some Target stores.

Stevia: Stevia is a plant native to South America, and you can even grow it yourself. As awareness of the dangers of artificial sweeteners has increased, stevia has become more popular. Be sure to read labels, however, because a product that is advertised as stevia may have harmful ingredients mixed in. Stevia is extremely sweet, but has an aftertaste. I like it; my husband hates it. Pure stevia is usually only found in health food stores, but recently my local grocery store started carrying a brand called Stevia in the Raw.

Stevia blends: Stevia is sometimes combined with Xyletol, which is also safe. Most grocery stores now carry a product

A Web site that ranks sweeteners on the glycemic index is: www.fitsugar.com/3031565.

You may want to consider reading *Eat, Cheat and Melt the Fat Away* by Suzanne Somers. It has a glycemic index on page 81. It also has great recipes and more information on insulin resistance and hormone imbalance.

Here's a good Web site about agave nectar: www.allaboutagave.com.

called Purevia, which I like. Purevia has a cleaner taste than pure stevia. This product mixes stevia with Erythritol and Isomaltulose. Erythritol is a sugar alcohol, and Isomaltulose is a sugar enzyme.

SomerSweet: This product was developed by Suzanne Somers and can only be purchased through her Web site. This product is five times sweeter than sugar and is very tasty. It works well in most recipes, but not all, so it takes some experimentation. Baked goods seem to come out dry and a little crumbly.

The original SomerSweet contains small amounts of acesulfame K (Ace K). Ace K has been studied and approved as safe in Europe, which has stricter regulations on food safety than the United States. However, some United States companies—mostly the soda industry and the artificial sweetener industry—have generated some controversy over Ace K. If you are concerned about the Ace K in the original SomerSweet, you can try a new, all-natural SomerSweet. This product has a clean, mildly sweet taste. Although Suzanne advertises it as being equivalent in sweetness to white sugar, I find it less sweet. This product also becomes caked very easily.

SODAS

One important step you can take to decrease your risk of cancer is to stop drinking sodas. Diet sodas are loaded with toxic sugar substitutes. Regular sodas are mainly sugar. Both contain toxic petro-chemicals.

EAT HEALTHY FATS AND OILS

We've often been warned about too much fat in our diets. That warning is half right. Our bodies require certain fats in order to survive. Especially our brains. So, the advice to eliminate fats from our diets is dangerous. This advice, which created the low-fat craze, has also led to a higher sugar intake. The advice should be to eliminate all bad fats from our diets. A "bad fat" is a fat that is high in omega-6 fatty acids. Omega-6 fatty acids are unhealthy because they:

- Suppress the immune system
- Are pro-inflammatory
- Stimulate cancer growth and spread

Here is the Web site for Somersweet:
www.suzannesomers.com.

- Impair cell function
- Increase damage to brain cells

The fats you should eat are "good fats" that are high in omega-3 fatty acids. Omega-3 fatty acids do the exact opposite of all those things listed above.

Good fats come from whole foods like nuts, vegetables, seeds, whole grains, deep water fish, and free-range eggs. Extra virgin olive oil and flaxseed oil are good fats. (Flaxseed oil should not be used, however, for cooking.) Bad fats can come from red meats and dairy but can also come from certain plants. Red meats (beef, pork, lamb) and chicken contain a cancer-promoting chemical called arachidonic acid. This acid is a by-product of the omega-6 fatty acid.

All synthetic fats, called trans fats, usually labeled "hydrogenated," are bad and should be avoided. These fats have been altered in order to turn the liquid fat into a solid in order to keep it from oxidizing quickly and thus extend the shelf life of a food product. The dangers of these fats are becoming common knowledge, as evidenced by all the "zero trans fats" labels showing up on products.

Processed foods that contain high amounts of omega-6 fatty acids are cakes, cookies, crackers, and chips.

Fats that are high in omega-6 fatty acids and should be avoided are corn, sunflower, safflower, peanut, soybean, and canola oils. (Canola oil has the lowest amount of omega-6 of all of these oils.) These fats all promote inflammation in your body. You want to avoid creating inflammation in your body because if your immune system is busy fighting inflammation, it may be too overworked to catch and destroy those cancer cells. If you already have an inflammatory condition such as arthritis or allergies, I suggest you take a supplement called Curcumin. This is derived from the spice tumeric and fights inflammation. I take 500 mg two times a day even though I am not aware of having any inflammatory conditions. While undergoing breast reconstruction, I was concerned that the implants might cause mild inflammation.

TRY THE BUDWIG PROTOCOL

In my research I discovered something called the Budwig Protocol, which is based on flaxseed oil. Many cancer patients

For more information on the Budwig Protocol, visit: www.cancertutor.com/Cancer/Budwig/html.

swear by it. I think the smoothies are fantastic, certainly can't hurt you, and are a good replacement for less healthy foods. The Budwig Protocol, developed by German scientist Dr. Johanna Budwig, combines flaxseed oil with either cottage cheese (preferred) or yogurt. If you like them, these smoothies are a simple step toward healthy eating.

MEAT AND DAIRY

In *Anti-Cancer: A New Way Of Life*, David Servan-Schreiber, MD, cited a twelve-year study of 91,000 nurses at Harvard University revealing that women who ate red meat more than once a day doubled their risk of breast cancer.

Because meat and dairy products are mainly fats, and toxins are stored in highest concentrations in fats, any toxins ingested by those animals are passed on down the food chain to you and then stored in your fats.

One of the riskiest hormones used in the food industry is Recombinant Bovine Growth Hormone (rBGH), and it is used in most non-organic dairy production in the United States. Developed by Monsanto Corporation, rBGH, contains high levels of a growth factor called IGF-1. IGF-1 has been linked to breast cancer and other cancers. Pasteurization does not destroy IGF-1. The food industry has successfully hidden this information from consumers in the United States. However, all meat and dairy from the United States that contains growth hormones has been banned in most other industrialized countries.

Due to pressure from breast cancer groups, Dannon and Yoplait will no longer be using milk with rBGH in their yogurt beginning in 2010. Costco already carries MountainHigh, an organic yogurt with no rBGH.

Women with ER+ or PR+ cancer often receive a prescription for Tamoxifen or Evista (estrogen blockers) and advice to avoid eating soy. While soy does contain estrogens, they are phytoestrogens (meaning plant-based) and water soluble, so they are easily excreted from the body. These women are better served by learning about and avoiding the dangerous fat-soluble fake estrogens in many other foods, such as meat and dairy products.

In the most comprehensive study ever done on nutrition, presented in the book *The China Study*, by T. Colin Campbell, PhD, and Thomas M. Campbell II, it was discovered that a diet that includes more than 10 percent in animal protein causes cancer to grow. Vegetable protein, even at much higher levels, did not have that same effect.

For more information about factory-style meat and dairy production, watch the movie *Food, Inc.*

For purposes of full disclosure, I need to reveal that I have been a vegetarian for more than twenty years. I do eat moderate amounts of organic milk, cheese, and eggs. And I think eating moderate amounts of organic, grass-fed meat and organic dairy can be part of a healthy diet. I chose to become a vegetarian at the time when meat and dairy became an industry in this country, no longer produced on the family farm but instead in large factory-style confinement buildings. Because meat and dairy produced in this factory-style environment must be dosed with antibiotics, fed cheap food, and often given growth hormones to fatten them up for market quickly, I decided that was simply not what I wanted to put into my body.

Organic meat and dairy are more expensive, and in some parts of the country, harder to find. I like milk and cheese more than meat. Because I couldn't afford to buy both, I chose to give up meat and to buy organic dairy and eggs. Once consumers start demanding more organic meat and dairy, however, more will be produced and the law of supply-and-demand will bring prices down.

Despite the constitutional right to freedom of speech, it is risky to speak truthfully about foods such as meat, poultry, or dairy. It's risky because some laws protect the meat, poultry, dairy, and other food industries. Lawsuits filed under these special protection laws are known as Strategic Lawsuits Against Public Participation (SLAPP). Oprah discovered SLAPP following her offhand remark about not wanting to eat hamburger after seeing how it was "produced." These laws prevent you from finding out not only how your food is produced, but also what you are really eating. Because I don't have big lawyers behind me, I have walked carefully through food topics above. For more in-depth information, please check the resources listed on this page.

EAT VEGETABLES AND FRUITS

Studies show that cancer rates are lower in populations that eat mostly fruits and vegetables. The reason: besides being loaded with vitamins, fruits and vegetables contain flavonoids. Flavonoids are a group of 5,000 different complex plant chemicals. Many of these flavonoids have been well-studied and identified as having antioxidants that have cancer-preventing abilities.

More information about rBGH is available at: www.organicconsumers.org/articles/article_3717.cfm.

Here's a helpful book about rBGH: *What's in Your Milk?* by Samuel S. Epstein, MD, with introduction by Ben Cohen, co-founder of Ben & Jerry's Ice Cream.

I found this Web site to contain important information about cancer prevention: www.preventcancer.com.

Here's an interesting book to read: *Righteous Porkchop* by Nocolette Hahn Niman.

For more information about SLAPP, see: www.prwatch. org/prwissues/1997q2/ slapp.html.

For information on genetically modified foods, watch the movie, *The Future of Food.*

For the dangers of eating fast foods, watch, *Supersize Me.*

These flavonoids work by also being able to inhibit the growth-related enzymes created by cancer cells.

Eat as many vegetables as you can, preferably organic and raw or steamed. Fruits are healthy, but they are also high in sugar, so eat more vegetables than fruits. The darker the fruit (all berries) the better. Fruit juice is not a substitute for eating fresh fruit because all the fiber is taken out and you are left with the sugars. Frozen berries are great in smoothies when fresh ones are not in season.

Besides eating vegetables and fruits, you can also drink them. Many people have juicers and think that juicing fruits and vegetables is healthy. While it may be healthier than not eating fruits and veggies at all, juicing leaves behind the all-important fiber and many nutrients, so is not a good choice. Blenderizing, on the other hand, includes all of the fiber and nutrients and is therefore very healthy. In fact, some doctors believe that drinking blended vegetable drinks each day will help prevent cancer. To blend whole raw fruits and vegetables you must have a special blender powerful enough to blend them into a drinkable consistency. I have the Vita Mix 5200, which works great. I also recently saw an infomercial by Montel Williams, who has developed a blender that appears to be as powerful as the Vita Mix at about half the price.

When you prepare your blended vegetable drink, do not just include all the fruits and vegetables that you like. Below is a list of possible ingredients, from *Natural Strategies For Cancer Patients* by Dr. Russell Blaylock. Choose at least five vegetables and two fruits for each batch of drink you blenderize. Use organic if possible, and always wash produce before you blenderize it. Add one cup of filtered water to the vegetables. If you have not been eating enough fiber, the blenderized vegetable drink may cause diarrhea or bloating at first. If this is a problem, start by drinking a mixture of half vegetable juice and half purified water. Eventually you want to drink 100 percent vegetable juice. You may also find it a chore to blenderize vegetables on a daily basis. In this case, blend a large batch and freeze individual daily portions (a 10–ounce glass twice a day).

If you find the taste too bitter, you can add spices such as fennel, basil, cilantro, or others that appeal to you. Spices contain beneficial plant flavonoids, too.

VEGETABLES

- Beets
- Carrots
- Broccoli
- Brussels Sprouts
- Celery
- Cauliflower
- Kale
- Parsley
- Purple Cabbage
- Spinach
- Tomatoes
- Turnip Greens

FRUITS

- Blueberries
- Blackberries
- Cranberries
- Strawberries
- Grapefruit
- McIntosh apples
- Oranges
- Raspberries
- Red currants

One easy way to start with improving a diet, is to increase your intake of the top ten anti-breast cancer foods—all of them vegetables. In *Foods That Fight Cancer*, Richard Beliveau says those top foods are the following:

- Garlic
- Leeks
- Scallions
- Brussels sprouts
- Cauliflower
- Cabbage
- Kale
- Broccoli
- Radishes
- Savoy cabbage

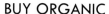

BUY ORGANIC

Why buy organic?

- Because organic fruits and vegetables are grown without the use of toxic pesticides and herbicides.
- Because meat from organically raised poultry and livestock does not contain growth hormones, and their feed was also organic and pesticide-free.
- Because whatever those animals ate goes into our bodies when we eat meat and dairy.
- Because buying and eating organic food reduces the toxins that accumulate in breast tissue.

In *What Your Doctor May Not Tell You About Breast Cancer*, Dr. John R. Lee cites an important clinical study by Mary Wolff of the Mount Sinai Medical Center in New York reported in the *Journal of the National Cancer Institute*. The study indicates that by mimicking estrogens (as xenoestrogens), pesticides could increase the risk of breast cancer by as much as 400 percent! Her study found that women who had breast cancer had at least 35 percent more DDE (which comes from the banned pesticide DDT) in their blood. Women with the highest levels of this pesticide residue had a breast cancer rate four times that of other women. While there are many critics who say pesticides don't cause cancer, Mary Wolff's study is not alone. Similar studies have been done recently in Finland, Connecticut, Hawaii, Israel, and other countries that have found similar connections between pesticide use and breast cancer.

More information about these pesticide studies and xeno-estrogens can be found in *It's My Ovaries Stupid!* by Elizabeth Lee Vliet, MD.

The non-organic ten fruits and vegetables with highest levels of pesticides are:

- Strawberries
- Bell Peppers
- Spinach
- Cherries (US grown)
- Peaches
- Celery
- Apples
- Green Beans

- Pears
- Raspberries

SPICES

It's a simple and flavorful step: start cooking with more spices. Spices are antioxidants, and they also contain plant flavonoids. Both are essential to our health, and many have specific cancer-fighting properties. In addition, your food tastes better!

Some spices that have specific cancer-fighting benefits are tumeric, oregano, ginger, rosemary, garlic, and chili peppers.

My favorite spices are often used in Indian and Mediterranean (Greek, Lebanese) cooking. Many places in the United States offer cooking classes featuring foods from different cultures. If you're new at this and the number of spices in your spice cabinet is less than a dozen, then buy some good cookbooks that explain how to use spices and that have simple recipes to follow. Better yet, get your girlfriends together for a day or weekend and take a cooking class. Choose one that features healthy eating and use of beneficial spices. You'll be hooked. If you are already an accomplished cook, go wild and be more experimental!

Amazon's book search function can help you find cookbooks using spices, especially if you read the customer reviews before ordering. Search especially for cookbooks on Indian, Mexican, and Asian cooking.

CURCUMIN, RESVERATROL, AND GREEN TEA

One spice that may have special value is tumeric, a spice used in curries. Along with being anti-inflammatory, it contains a special catechin called curcumin. Catechins, which are special plant flavonoids found also in green tea and red wine, prevent the growth of cancer cells by inhibiting something called Nuclear Factor Kappa B (NF-Kappa B).

Much scientific research is currently focused on NF-Kappa B because the growth and spread of cancer cells rely heavily on this pro-inflammatory agent. NF-Kappa B is not only resistant to many chemotherapy treatments, but is also activated by chemotherapy. Albert Baldwin, PhD and professor at the University of North Carolina, says, "Almost every cancer preventative is an

For more specific pesticide data, visit: www.organicconsumers. org/organic/pesticide-residues.cfm.

Here are two Web sites you can visit to learn more about NF-Kappa B:

www.cytok.com/showabstract.php?pmid=16243823&redirect=yes&terms=nf-kappa+b+and+breast+cancer

www.ncbi.nlm.nih.gov/pubmed/16728586?dopt=AbstractPlus

inhibitor of NF-Kappa B." So the search is on to create a patent able drug to block or inhibit NF-Kappa B.

But the substances known to inhibit NF-Kappa B are readily available in curcumin, (from tumeric) in red wine (as Resveratrol), and green tea! Tumeric, which must be mixed with pepper and oil, is available at most grocery stores and all Indian food stores. Curcumin, Resveratrol, and green tea extract can all be purchased in supplement form. Loose green tea must be steeped for five to ten minutes and drunk within an hour of steeping or the essential catechins lose their potency.

WATER

Drinking six to eight eight-ounce glasses of water every day helps our bodies flush out toxins. But that can't just be any water. Most municipal drinking water has toxins in it, chlorine and fluoride being the most common. Bottled water often isn't much better: plastic bottles are made from petroleum-based chemicals that get into the water. These chemicals are toxic xenoestrogens. Only filtered water, properly filtered by a process called reverse osmosis, is really beneficial. You can have a reverse osmosis water filtration system installed in your home. It is not cheap, but the cost of buying bottled water over time far exceeds the cost of installing your own filter.

Drinking six to eight glasses of water per day is not easy for me. I simply don't like plain water. I have two tricks to make water more appealing. I squeeze lemon juice (from a real lemon, not the plastic one) into a glass of filtered ice water and add a little stevia. Lemon juice has the additional benefit of helping change my body pH from acidic to alkaline, which is great because cancer requires an acidic environment to grow. This may seem contradictory since lemon juice is acidic. Although acidic in their natural state, orange juice and lemon juice both become alkaline once metabolized by the body. My second trick is making and refrigerating in a glass container huge batches of Celestial Seasonings Herbal Teas in a flavor I like (I love the Berry Zingers or Mango Acai Zinger). You can sweeten these teas if you like with any of the good artificial sweeteners recommended above. These teas also do not contain caffeine.

STORE FOOD IN GLASS CONTAINERS

Avoid storing foods in plastic containers because most are made from petrochemicals, which release toxins into their contents. Plastic #7 releases BPA (bisphenal A), plastic #1 releases Phthalates, plastic #3 releases dioxins, and plastic #6 (Styrofoam) releases styrenes. All of these are toxic to our bodies and most have been linked to cancer. I can't remember all those numbers so I simply use glass containers instead. I went to thrift stores and bought glass containers to replace all of my plastics.

Never reuse plastic containers that you buy food or water in because those are intended for single-use only. If reused, they leach the harmful petrochemical toxins listed above into your food. Many women wonder about products such as Tupperware that are intended for multiple use and food storage. Some of these products are made from plastics that are safe—but not all. Again, I can't remember all the numbers so it is simpler—and safer—to avoid as much plastic in contact with food as possible. Never microwave in plastic containers or using plastic wrap. And, of course, to be earth-friendly, recycle all plastic containers.

SHOP HEALTHY BY READING LABELS

The only way you are going to know what's really in your food is by reading labels—the labels in microscopic print on the back of the product, not the larger label that lists grams of fats, carbohydrates, sodium, protein, and sugars. The larger labels are misleading and don't tell you what's actually in that product. It's no coincidence that this label is larger and gets more attention than the microscopically printed list of ingredients.

Be especially wary of the terms "all natural" or "whole wheat" on the front of products. These words deceive you into thinking you are buying something healthy. A perfect example is an "all natural" granola or energy bar. Read the label on the back of those (any brand) and you'll find that they are mostly sugars (remember, dried fruit is mostly sugar).

Once you start reading the small labels, you will become aware of how poisoned our food supply is. Ingredients are listed in the order of the greatest to the least amounts. If the first ingredient listed is sugar, that product has more sugar than anything

This Web site provides more information about plastics, including a list of the Tupperware products made from "bad" plastics: http://life.gaiam.com/gaiam/p/Are-Plastic-Food-Containers-Safe-to-Reuse.html.

This Web site lists harmful and deceptive ingredients in foods: www.healthyeatingadvisor.com.

else in it. Sugar comes with many other names such as high fructose corn syrup, honey, molasses, brown rice syrup, fructose, and dried fruit. Organic sugar doesn't make it healthy either. And even if a toxic ingredient is last on the list, it is significant because toxins are stored in your body and accumulate. Over time, frequent ingestion of tiny amounts of toxins results in lots of toxins in your body and breast tissue.

Turn off your cell phone while grocery shopping! Think of how often you've seen a woman put items in a grocery cart while carrying on a phone conversation. This woman has no idea what she is putting into her cart and then into her body. You can't make good food choices if you don't read labels. You obviously can't read labels if you are talking on your cell phone.

GOOGLE SEARCH SUGGESTIONS

Toxins
- Toxins found in breast tissue
- Toxins cause breast cancer
- Pesticides and breast cancer
- Petrochemicals and cancer
- How to detoxify your body
- Antioxidants prevent cancer
- Glutathione and cancer prevention
- Glycemic Index (Print a copy and hang it on your refrigerator.)

Artificial sweeteners
- Is Splenda safe?
- Is Aspartame safe?
- Is NutraSweet safe?

rBGH
- Is rBGH safe?
- IGF-1 and breast cancer

Pesticides
- Pesticides in our food
- Pesticide levels in produce
- What is organic?
- Pesticides and breast cancer
- Are pesticides safe?

sSpices

- Cooking with spices
- Spices that fight cancer
- NF-Kappa B and breast cancer
- Resveratrol and breast cancer
- Curcumin and breast cancer
- Green tea and breast cancer

Miscellaneous

- Plastics and cancer
- Plastic food storage and cancer
- Bottled water and cancer
- What to watch for on food labels
- Dangers of drinking soda

If you have any doubts about how what you eat either causes or prevents cancer, I urge you to read *The China Study*, by T. Colin Campbell, PhD, and Thomas M. Campbell II.

For the first time in the history of the world, every human being is now subjected to contact with dangerous chemicals, from the moment of conception until death.

RACHEL CARSON, *SILENT SPRING*, 1962

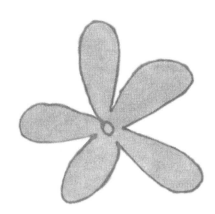

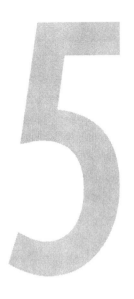

Prevention: Supplements and Lifestyle

Your immune system is on the front line, constantly fighting and killing invaders that seek to do you harm. This is the system responsible for ridding your body of damaged cells, cells that could eventually become cancer cells. Preventing breast cancer or a recurrence of breast cancer requires that you make your immune system as strong as possible. Avoiding toxins and eating a healthy diet are two areas that go a long way in fortifying your immune system. Supplements and certain lifestyle changes can also greatly enhance your immune system's ability to identify and kill damaged cells. If you've been diagnosed with breast cancer, specific supplements have been proven effective in preventing recurrence and metastases.

SUPPLEMENTS

Supplements are not a substitute for a good diet, rich in fruits and vegetables. They are, as their name implies, a supplement to a good diet, insurance for getting all the vitamins and minerals that your body needs to function properly. Supplements are vitamins and minerals in pill or liquid form. They boost our immune systems, and many are powerful antioxidants. Food today is less nutritious than it was decades ago, due to depleted soil, over-processing, and required transportation time. Quality vitamin and mineral supplements are a key to filling in the resulting nutritional gaps. Many also have very specific cancer preventive properties.

Vitamin and mineral supplements must be taken in the correct form, a form that your body can use. This means they must be bioavailable. If a vitamin is fat-soluble (meaning it requires a fat or an oil to be used by your cells), taking it in a dry pill form will do no good. Also, vitamins derived from natural sources, such as algae or yeasts, are often more beneficial than the synthetic versions because they contain all the essential components of that vitamin. I doubt that there is one multi-vitamin that will provide all the vitamins and minerals you need, in the proper amounts, and in the forms that your body can absorb. I searched and couldn't find it. You may find some good vitamin or mineral combinations, such as all of the B vitamins, in one supplement, but you will most likely have to take most vitamins or minerals as individual supplements.

Many health-conscious women have heard about the benefits of Vitamin D, CoQ10, and Vitamin E. However, if women receive this information piecemeal, some immediately start mega-dosing on one or two specific vitamins or minerals. Because vitamins and minerals work synergistically (together), taking just one or two supplements may actually cause more harm than good. And taking too much of any of them can be damaging.

The best resource I found for identifying which vitamins and minerals you need, and in which form, is Dr. Russell Blaylock's book, *Natural Strategies for Cancer Patients*. If you are receiving radiation or chemotherapy treatments, this book is essential! Refer to Dr. Blaylock's book for the best form of each supplement and dosage. Dosages will be different for a woman who has or has had breast cancer, or is undergoing radiation or chemotherapy than for a woman who wants to prevent breast cancer. This book also has an excellent resource section for help finding specific supplements.

These are the essential vitamins and minerals:
- Vitamin A*
- Vitamin B1, B2, B3, B5, B6, B12*
- Biotin
- Boron

In addition to Dr. Russell Blaylock's book, *Natural Strategies for Cancer Patients*, I recommend reading *Health and Nutrition Secrets*, also by Blaylock.

- Vitamin C*
- Calcium*
- Choline
- Chromium
- CoQ10
- Vitamin D
- Vitamin E*
- Folic Acid
- Vitamin K
- Magnesium*
- Manganese
- Molybdenum
- Omega-3 (fish oil capsules)
- Selenium
- Zinc

A study by Dr. Pamela Goodwin of Mount Sinai Medical Center in Toronto reveals that low levels of vitamin D have been linked to higher breast cancer risk and higher risk of recurrence. Most women have low levels of vitamin D and don't know it.

These supplements must be taken in a specific form in order to be absorbed by the body.

IRON

Iron is not on the essential vitamin list. An excess of iron actually creates an environment for cancer cells to grow. Without a known iron deficiency, taking iron supplements is risky.

SPECIFIC SUPPLEMENTS THAT FIGHT BREAST CANCER

Many studies have been done on the following list of supplements that have shown them to be active in both the prevention of breast cancer and in preventing recurrence or metastases. By doing a Google search on any of these you will find much more in-depth information including studies documenting the biological means by which they work against breast cancer. There are other supplements that work to make chemotherapy or radiation treatments more effective and alleviate their side effects.

To see a full report on Dr. Goodwin's study, visit: www.mountsinai.on.ca/care/mkbc/resources-2/mount-sinais-dr-pam-goodwin-reveals-vitamin-d-deficiency-associated-with-breast-cancer.

I earlier recommended reading Dr. Blaylock's book, *Natural Strategies for Cancer Patients.* It also discusses supplements that can be used to increase the effectiveness of chemotherapy and radiation treatments.

SULFORAPHANE

I encourage all women to research two products, BroccoMax (by Jarrow Formulas) and Oncoplex, especially if you have been diagnosed with breast cancer. Studies in animals and in humans are finding the essential ingredient sulforaphane (from broccoli sprouts) very promising in fighting breast cancer. This discovery was made by two scientists at Johns Hopkins Medical Center.

I was advised by a health care professional to take 30 mg four times a day for the first year following my mastectomy and after that to drop to a maintenance dose of 30 mg twice a day.

CURCUMIN

If you have any inflammation in your body, from arthritis, allergies, dental disease, or any other inflammatory condition, research suggests that taking curcumin (from the spice tumeric) fights inflammation. Fish oil also fights inflammation. As stated earlier, if your immune system is overworked fighting inflammation, then it can miss the cancer cells that it usually destroys.

BETA GLUCANS

If you have breast cancer, other supplements to research are Glucans: Beta 1, 3 and Beta 1, 6. These compounds are very effective in boosting your immune system. Beta Glucans are found in yeast, shiitake, maitaki, and reishi mushrooms, and in some seaweeds. Exact dosage and combinations are important, so study these in Dr. Russell Blaylock's book, *Natural Strategies for Cancer Patients*.

DIGESTIVE ENZYMES

One mechanism cancer cells use to evade your immune system is the creation of specific immune-blocking proteins. The cancer cells cloak themselves with these proteins so that your immune system doesn't recognize and destroy them as they travel through the digestive system. Digestive enzymes called proteolytic enzymes strip away these proteins, leaving the cancer cells exposed.

According to Dr. Blaylock, most digestive enzymes are sold with the instructions that they be taken with food. However, they only work to strip the proteins from cancer cells if taken on an empty stomach. If taken with food, they will be used instead to break down the proteins in the food. These enzymes also help reduce inflammation in all tissues, a reduction critical for cancer prevention. Note that proteolytic enzymes are not the same as probiotics, often found in yogurts.

MODIFIED CITRUS PECTIN

Modified citrus pectin is a water-soluble fiber used as cell cement in plants. According to Dr. Blaylock, in animal studies, the pectin appears to prevent metastasis by preventing the cancer cells from sticking to the walls of blood vessels. Modified citrus pectin comes in a powdered form. I blend it in my smoothies. Modified citrus pectin is not the same as fruit pectin used to make jams and jellies.

Caution: Do not purchase your supplements at discount stores. High-quality supplements are only found in health food stores and at some online sources.

IODINE

It appears that iodine deficiency may be a major risk factor for breast cancer. A must-read is the book, *Iodine: Why You Need It and Why You Can't Live Without It*, by the noted expert on iodine, Dr. David Brownstein. He explains that in women, besides the thyroid gland, one of the places iodine is stored is in the breasts. If we are deficient in iodine, the thyroid gland will "steal" what it needs from the breasts, leaving them deficient and vulnerable to fibrocystic tumors and cancer. Another author concurs. In his book *Breast Cancer and Iodine: How to Prevent and Survive Breast Cancer*, David Derry, MD, PhD, explains how breast cancer metastasizes first to the connective tissues before invading organs or bones. Adequate iodine and thyroid hormone appear to stop the cancer cells from moving beyond the connective tissue. He also explains that the presence of iodine is necessary for cell apoptosis (cell death) and that a lack of iodine may be one of the reasons cancer cells do not undergo apoptosis and instead continue to grow. Both authors also point out the

While researching herbal supplements, I discovered a wonderful Web site set up by Memorial Sloan-Kettering Cancer Center. This Web site provides information on effectiveness and side effects, and a full list of additional studies on almost all herbal supplements. The easiest way to find this site is to Google search: mskcc about herbs.

For information about ordering supplements, visit this Web site: www.iherb.com.

connection between iodine deficiency and increased estrogen, another known breast cancer risk factor.

While the importance of iodine in our diet was recognized years ago, which led to salt being iodized, the RDA (recommended daily allowance) of iodine is only sufficient to prevent goiters and cretinism; it is not sufficient to maintain a healthy body. In America, we have few if any sources of iodine in our diet other than iodized salt.

Iodine is utilized by every cell in our body. We need enough iodine to saturate the thyroid gland and the breasts and to circulate throughout our bodies. It takes approximately 6 mg of iodine a day just to saturate the thyroid gland. The female breasts need approximately 5 mg of iodine a day. Average Americans get less than a few mg a day from their diet, mainly from iodized salt. That is not even enough to saturate the thyroid gland. So, we need more than 11 mg a day in order to have enough to reach all the cells in our bodies. Japanese women, who have the world's lowest rate of breast cancer, get 10 to 13 mg of iodine a day in their diet, which is high in seaweed and fish, both major sources of iodine. Once Japanese women move to the United States and eat the typical American diet, their iodine intake decreases, and they eventually have breast cancer rates equal to American women.

It is interesting to note that breast feeding is known to reduce a woman's risk of breast cancer. While lactating, iodine is concentrated in the breast tissue thirty times higher than in the rest of the body. It appears that iodine is protective to the breast tissue.

If you have fibrocystic breasts, you should definitely do some research on iodine.

Iodine deficiency has been linked to fibrocystic breasts, and there is now a great deal of evidence that fibrocystic breasts are a precursor to DCIS and breast cancer. Clinical trials show that taking an iodine supplement called Iodoral (this is the pill form of Lugol's Iodine) which combines iodine and iodide, will cause fibrocystic disease to dissolve.

Besides not taking in enough iodine, we do many things that actually cause what little iodine we have to be depleted. Diets high in fat deplete the body of iodine. Nitrates, found in unfiltered drinking water, non-organic fruits and vegetables,

Here's a Web site that provides more information on iodine deficiency as it may relate to breast cancer: www.breastcancerchoices.org. You can also order Iodoral (a safe iodine supplement) from this Web site.

and food preservatives block the uptake of iodine by the thyroid gland. Bromine (found in many breads) and fluoride also block the absorption of iodine. Iodine supplementation appears to be a critical element in breast cancer prevention.

Interestingly, in men iodine deficiency can lead to prostate cancer, because men concentrate iodine in their prostate. Japanese men have one of the lowest rates of prostate cancer and highest intake of iodine.

In his practice, Dr. Brownstein found that nearly 95 percent of his patients were iodine-deficient and those women with breast cancer had the highest deficiencies. It is important to find out if you have an iodine deficiency. This cannot be determined by your T3 and T4 levels on a hormone test. The proper test to determine if you are iodine-deficient is called an iodine loading test. It is a 24-hour urine test. There are only a few labs in this country that perform this test. I recommend using FFP Laboratory, owned and operated by Dr. Jorge D. Flechas, another expert on iodine. At the time of this printing, the cost for the iodine spot test (establishes a baseline) and the 24-hour iodine loading test was $117. This includes a phone consultation about the results with Dr. Flechas.

COSMETICS

Skin absorbs everything put onto it, so putting something on your skin has the same impact as eating it—a good reason that cosmetics should be as toxin-free as food. Personal care products do not need FDA approval for safety. The National Institute for Occupational Health lists 884 chemicals used in personal care products as being toxins. The European Union has banned 450 chemicals from use in these products, but they are still allowed in the United States. The Campaign for Safe Cosmetics has gotten over 300 companies to voluntarily rid their products of these toxic chemicals. A few of those companies are L'Oreal, Revlon, Avalon, and Unilever.

Mary Kay, Avon, Arbonne, Melaleuca, and Nu Skin are a few companies not willing to remove the toxins. Some cosmetic companies hypocritically place the breast cancer pink ribbon on products containing cancer-causing ingredients. Many of these chemicals are known carcinogens (cause cancer) and some are xenoestrogens (meaning they act like estrogens in the body).

Dr. Flechas' Web site is: www.iodine4health.com. The phone number is 1-877-900-5556.

Here's another Web site with information about the iodine test, the lab, and Dr. Flechas: www.breastcancerchoices.org. Search under iodine testing.

Here are some Web sites about toxins in cosmetics and other personal-care products:

www.safecosmetics.org

www.ewg.org (Search under skin deep.)

www.thinkbeforeyoupink.org

www.skinbiology.com

www.notjustaprettyface.org

www.thegreenbeautyguide.com

www.envirocancer.cornell.edu/research/endocrine/videos/makeup.cfm#screens

And, here are some books that tell more about toxins and cosmetics:

Don't Go To The Cosmetics Counter Without Me, 7th edition, by Paula Begoun

Drop Dead Gorgeous: Protecting Yourself from the Hidden Dangers of Cosmetics by Kim Erickson

Toxic Beauty: How Cosmetics and Personal Care Products Endanger Your Health and What You Can Do About It by Samuel S. Epstein, MD, and Randall Fitzgerald

Reading cosmetic labels, like reading food labels, may save your breasts.

There are many toxic chemicals found in personal care products. Below are some of the worst:

- Sodium Laurel Sulfate: This is found in almost all shampoos and in many other products. It easily penetrates the skin and accumulates in the heart, liver, lungs, and brain. It can become carcinogenic when mixed with other chemicals.
- Propylene Glycol: This is a highly toxic chemical that causes brain, kidney, and liver damage. It is found in some anti-perspirants and in hair-care products.
- DEA, MEA and TEA: These are hormone-disrupting and cancer-causing chemicals. They are found in shampoos and body wash.
- Dibutyl Phthalate: This chemical has been banned in Europe because it causes cancer. It is most commonly found in nail polish, but may also be found in hairspray and anti-perspirant.
- Artificial Colors: These are found in many make-up products such as lipsticks, nail polish, and eye shadows. Blue #1 and Green #3 are carcinogenic, as are any colors with FD & C pigments (which are made from coal tar).
- Formaldehyde: This is a preservative that weakens the immune system, damages the respiratory system, and causes cancer. High levels are found in nail polishes.
- Parabens: This includes any ingredient ending in –paraben. These chemicals mimic estrogens (xenoestrogens) which can increase your risk of breast cancer. Parabens are found in many personal-care products.
- Benzophenones (Oxybenzone): This chemical is used in most sunscreens as a UV absorber and filter. It is easily absorbed into the body and accumulates in body tissue. It causes cellular changes with long-term effects yet unknown.
- Placental extracts: Yes, these are exactly what the name says. These extracts are high in hormones, especially estrogens, that are easily absorbed into the bloodstream. Placental extracts are found in skin creams and hair conditioners.

Concern is increasing about a link between aluminum found in anti-perspirants and breast cancer. Aluminum from anti-perspirants is definitely absorbed into the breasts, but the question is whether it can cause cancer. Benign breasts cysts have been shown to contain high levels of aluminum, and the most likely source is anti-perspirants. Aluminum-free anti-perspirants can be found at health food stores or online.

For information about aluminum-free anti-perspirants, visit: www.iherb.com.

OVER-THE-COUNTER AND PRESCRIPTION DRUGS

Many people in the United States are taking legal drugs they don't need; this includes both prescription and over-the-counter medications. Pharmaceutical companies' marketing campaigns and television ads convince people that drugs can fix every problem they have, and—even worse—that they have a problem they don't really have. Under pressure from their patients and drug companies, doctors write unnecessary prescriptions every day. And drugs rarely cure illness; they simply mask symptoms. Yes, under certain circumstances drugs are necessary, but drugs are chemical substances with profound consequences in your body—all drugs have side effects. So it's a trade-off. While a certain drug may stop your hot flashes and mood swings during menopause, it can also give you breast cancer. This is the trade-off for Prempro and other estrogen pills and patches that have been widely prescribed for women. Certain antidepressant drugs can actually double a woman's risk of breast cancer. Research published in the *British Journal of Cancer*, found that certain tricyclic antidepressants caused DNA damage in laboratory experiments. These antidepressants are sold under the brand names Asendin, Anafranil, Norpramin, Surmontil, Rhotrimine, and Paxil. All drugs have a good and bad side. Unfortunately, patients usually hear only the good side.

Information on this study on antidepressants is available at: www.prozactruth.com/cancer.htm.

Information on this study is also available at: www.abcnews.go.com/print?id=7716343.

In addition, the more drugs that are taken, the harder it is to predict the side effects of their interaction. Doctors are not well-informed about negative side effects of a single drug, let alone the dangerous drug cocktails that most Americans are taking. It now appears that taking certain antidepressant drugs, called SSRI's (selective serotonin reuptake inhibitors) in combination with the drug tamoxifen, actually inhibits the enzyme CYP2D6. This enzyme helps the body process tamoxifen, a drug widely prescribed for women with estrogen receptor positive breast cancer.

Drugs can also deplete important vitamins and minerals from your body, weakening your immune system. Talk with your doctor about the level of need for any drugs you are taking.

The bottom line is that all drugs are toxic substances and should be avoided unless absolutely necessary because we don't really know the full effect they have on our bodies. According to Dr. Janet Woodcock, a top Food and Drug Administration (FDA) official, it can take a hundred years for all the risks of a drug to be known.

The best policy is to take as few prescription and over-the-counter drugs as possible. You should work with your doctor to get off any prescription drugs that are not absolutely essential. When my doctor whips out the prescription pad, I ask two questions:

- Will my body naturally heal itself without the drugs?
- Is there a more natural remedy that can fix this problem?

For me, other than pain relief after surgery or an antibiotic for a serious infection, the answer to those two questions has almost always been yes. So, I have said no to most prescription drugs because I don't really need them.

STRESS

It's hard to underestimate the damage that stress can do to a body. By raising cortisol (a hormone) levels, stress depresses your immune system. And chronically elevated levels of cortisol have been linked to breast cancer—along with Alzheimer's disease, osteoporosis, high blood pressure, and weight gain.

Chronic stress not only depresses your immune system, it also increases the formation of free radicals, making it a double whammy. I know from experience that having breast cancer and trying to figure out the best treatment for yourself is stressful. But proper diet, exercise, and adequate sleep can alleviate stress. (See Chapter 6 for more details about cortisol, hormones, and stress.)

SLEEP

When I became perimenopausal, I began have difficulty sleeping through the night—a common complaint among

For further reading, check out Our Daily Meds by Melody Petersen.

menopausal women. Because getting seven to eight hours of sleep each night is critical to a healthy immune system, sleeplessness must be addressed.

Taking sleeping pills is not the answer because they do not induce the deep levels of sleep that your body needs in order to rejuvenate. Melatonin does.

We naturally produce melatonin, a hormone that makes us sleep. But as we age, most of us produce less and less of it. So, the simple, safe, and effective natural solution is to take 3 mg of melatonin an hour before you go to bed. Once I started taking melatonin, I was able to sleep soundly through the night. Be careful not to take more than 3 mg because an increased dose may cause heart palpitations. If you have a heart condition, talk to your doctor first.

EXERCISE

Regular, moderate exercise has been shown to lower the risk of breast cancer. Exercise works against cancer by improving your immune system and by oxygenating your tissues (cancer hates oxygen). You don't have to go to a gym to exercise. Moderate exercising includes brisk walking, bike riding, weight training, aerobics, Pilates, and yoga. I have been doing yoga regularly for six years, and I attribute my fast recovery from my mastectomy to my yoga practice, and so do my doctors. Yoga is also a great stress reliever.

MAMMOGRAMS

A mammogram is not a form of breast cancer prevention; it is a form of detection, but not always a reliable one. Although mammograms can detect many breast cancers before they get to a size that can be felt by self-exam, that is not always the case. I felt my 6 mm lump in my left breast because it was located near the surface of my skin. It had not shown up on my mammogram five months earlier, and it did not show up on the mammogram I had after I detected it.

Both of my mammograms used the newer digital technology. In addition, the 6 mm invasive cancer nodule that was later discovered in that same breast was not detected in either mammogram or on a more sensitive test called an MRI. My

As mentioned in the previous chapter, here is a good Web site for further information: www.preventcancer.com.

breast cancer was not the extremely aggressive type that grow rapidly. The tumors existed when those tests were done; the test simply did not detect them.

Women should not be lulled into a false sense of security by annual mammograms. Obviously, not all tumors show up on mammograms, and some mammograms can be especially hard to read due to dense breast tissue, breast implants, or damage from radiation treatments. Eshan Samei, of the Advanced Imaging Laboratory at Duke University Medical Center, estimates the average diagnostic error in reading medical images is 20-30 percent.

Some doctors believe that routine mammograms may actually increase a woman's risk of breast cancer by repeated exposure to radiation. Radiation exposure is a known carcinogen. The question becomes: how much radiation is too much? Some doctors are actually recommending against the routine annual mammogram unless there is reason for concern. I am not sure I would go that far, but I do want to warn women that mammograms are not prevention and should not be used as an excuse for not taking other measures to reduce your risk of breast cancer.

GOOGLE SEARCH SUGGESTIONS

- Dr. Pam Goodwin Vitamin D
- Oncoplex and breast cancer
- Studies on Sulforaphane and breast cancer
- Studies on curcumin and inflammation
- Beta Glucans and cancer prevention
- Iodine and fibrocystic breasts
- Iron levels and cancer
- Iodine and breast cancer
- Dr. Brownstein and iodine
- Dr. David Derry and iodine
- Iodine and fibrocystic breasts
- Dr. Guy Abraham and iodine
- Are cosmetics safe?
- Cancer causing ingredients in cosmetics
- Pink Ribbon campaign and cosmetics
- Cosmetics cause breast cancer
- Melatonin for sleep

- Are mammograms safe?
- Radiation from mammograms and cancer risks
- Can mammograms cause cancer?
- Does early detection of breast cancer lead to longer life?

An excellent magazine to subscribe to for information on healthy eating, lifestyle, and beneficial supplements is *Body and Soul*. It can be found at www. bodyandsoulmag.com.

Facts do not cease to exist because they are ignored.

ALDOUS HUXLEY

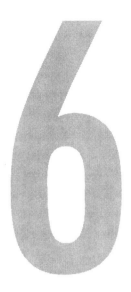

Hormones: The Elephant in the Room

Because hormones govern so many important functions and systems in our bodies, it is crucial for good health and disease prevention that all the hormones be at their correct levels and functioning synergistically (together). Hormone levels that are too high or too low (imbalanced) lead to a decrease or impairment of function and eventual breakdown of vital organs and the immune system. Many diseases, such as diabetes, depression, obesity, heart problems, autoimmune diseases, and cancers, are ultimately due to hormonal imbalances. Hormonal imbalances can be caused by stress, emotional issues, poor diet, and toxins. Good health requires that our hormones are in balance.

Hormones and hormonal imbalance are rarely mentioned as factors in the cause and prevention of breast cancer. So much research has been done that has proven the link between hormones (especially estrogen) and an increased risk of breast cancer, that it is unbelievable that not all doctors recognize the symptoms of hormonal imbalance and treat them before they manifest into serious health problems such as breast cancer. These symptoms appear in women long before their breast cancer gets started.

If you are over forty, and take only one step to prevent breast cancer, it should be to take a hormone level test by a doctor or

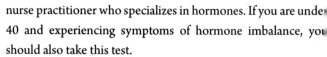

nurse practitioner who specializes in hormones. If you are under 40 and experiencing symptoms of hormone imbalance, you should also take this test.

Along with the hormones our bodies naturally produce, we are bombarded by hormone imitators called xenoestrogens in the form of toxic chemicals in our food, water, and cosmetics. Some doctors feel that increased exposure to these xenoestrogens is the reason that the age of female puberty in the United States is now two years earlier than it was just twenty years ago. Early menstruation is a well-established risk factor for breast cancer because the earlier a woman starts menstruating, the longer her body is exposed to estrogen. An earlier onset of puberty heralds a higher rate of breast cancer to come.

What are we talking about when we say hormones? Most of us just think of the sex hormones, estrogen and testosterone, but our body produces and relies on other important hormones to function. Because they all work together, they must all be in balance for a body to be free of disease.

HORMONES IN BRIEF

- Estrogen: Estrogen is not a single hormone, but a group of three hormones:
  - Estrone (E1): Produced by the adrenal glands and fat cells. Highest levels after menopause.
  - Estradiol (E2): Produced mainly by the ovaries. Stimulates growth in breast and uterine tissue. Predominant before menopause. High levels linked to breast cancer.
  - Estriol (E3): Reaches its highest level during pregnancy. Produced from estrone and estradiol and is the least stimulating to breast tissue. Women with higher estriol levels tend to have lower rates of breast cancer.
- Progesterone: Produced primarily in the ovaries and in small quantities by the adrenal glands. Protects against breast cancer.
- Testosterone: Produced in the ovaries and by the adrenal glands. Promotes muscle mass, bone density, well-being, and healing.
- DHEA: Secreted by the adrenal glands. Stimulates the immune system, decreases cholesterol and body fat. Es-

trogens and testosterone are made from DHEA.

- Pregnenolone: Produced in the adrenal glands as well as the brain, liver, and ovaries. It is a precursor to DHEA and progesterone. Appears to promote proper brain function.
- Thyroid: A group of hormones that regulate metabolism. The two main thyroid hormones are T3 and T4. T3, the active thyroid hormone, is produced in the brain and liver via conversion of T4. T4 is produced by the thyroid gland and is inactive.
- Melatonin: Secreted by the pineal gland and affects sleep. Melatonin increases the deep levels of sleep needed to produce natural killer cells that enhance immunity.
- Cortisol (one of the corticosteroids): Made by the adrenal glands in response to stress. An imbalance in cortisol levels increases the risk of breast cancer.
- Insulin: The blood-sugar regulating hormone made in the pancreas.

Obviously, certain hormones have very specific effects on breast cancer risk. So, you would think that as women enter perimenopause or menopause, and go to their doctors with clear symptoms of hormonal imbalance such as weight gain, headaches, weepiness, loss of libido, memory loss, fibroid tumors, fibrocystic breasts, etc., that they would be tested and treated for those hormonal imbalances. When I went to see my doctor about my fibroid tumors, hormonal imbalance was never even discussed, even though it is the cause of fibroid tumors. In the survey conducted for this book, many of the women indicated that they had symptoms of hormonal imbalance long before their breast cancer diagnosis. Quite a few of these women were on standard Hormone Replacement Therapy (HRT), which meant they were taking synthetic hormones. Without ever testing their hormone levels in order to actually balance them, their doctors had simply given them a standard dose of synthetic hormones (estrogens, most likely).

HORMONES AND BREAST CANCER

The Food and Drug Administration (FDA) has now warned us about the use of synthetic hormones, and the World Health

To fully understand how hormone imbalances lead to breast cancer, and to spot the symptoms, I urge you to read Dr. John R. Lee's book, *What Your Doctor May Not Tell You About Breast Cancer.*

Organization lists these synthetic hormones as cancer-causing. Many doctors who are knowledgeable about hormones believe the increase in breast cancer rates in the United States over the last twenty years is a result of the wide use of these synthetic hormones to treat menopausal symptoms. In fact, once the link between the synthetic estrogen, Prempro, and breast cancer was widely publicized in 2002, the number of prescriptions for that drug dropped by 65 percent. Not coincidentally, the breast cancer rates that had been increasing steadily since its widespread use, dropped by an astonishing 7 percent only one year after the huge drop in women taking Prempro.

The discovery that synthetic hormones can cause breast cancer came twenty years after women started using them. There is still so much misunderstanding in the medical field regarding hormones that today, even if you have symptoms of hormonal imbalance, doctors will either simply refuse to prescribe hormones because they know the damage that synthetic hormones can do (synthetic hormones come under the labels Prempro or Premarin and are also in most birth control pills) or they will actually prescribe these harmful synthetic hormones.

Hormonal imbalances are a symptom that something is not working properly in your body; they are not the "disease" itself. When a patient with symptoms of hormonal imbalance visits a doctor, the correct medical practice should be 1) test all hormone levels, 2) uncover the cause of the hormonal imbalance, which is most often emotional and dietary, and 3) work to correct the situation that is creating the imbalance. Without this protocol, women either simply go untreated or are given the wrong hormones altogether and often in the wrong doses. For example, you may exhibit all the symptoms of low estrogen, but without a hormone test, your doctor can't know which of the three estrogens is low, or what is causing the deficiency. It could be that out-of-balance cortisol levels are the cause of the estrogen imbalance. Prescribing estrogen in this case would be disastrous. Simply slapping on an estrogen patch may actually be doing more damage than just increasing your breast cancer risk.

It is now well established that women taking synthetic hormones are at an increased risk for breast cancer. So what about bioidentical hormones? Are they safe? Most leading doctors who have actually used them and studied them feel they are safe to use if used in the correct dosage, and if closely monitored. However, it must be stated that few studies have been done on the long-term effects of bioidentical hormones, so no one can say for sure whether or not they are safe. Synthetic hormones were considered safe until twenty years of use proved they were not. If you mention testing and balancing your hormones to your doctor, especially if you have breast cancer, your doctor's eyes may widen with alarm. This reaction is mainly based on a lack of knowledge. Much information is available on hormonal imbalance and breast cancer, synthetic hormones, and bioidentical hormones, so I strongly urge you to do your own research on this subject. If you feel you may have a hormonal imbalance, your first step is to take a saliva hormone test to see if you have any imbalances in the first place.

BIOIDENTICAL HORMONES VS. SYNTHETIC HORMONES

The confusion between synthetic (molecularly altered) hormones, which do not match the hormones your body produces, and bioidentical hormones, which are molecularly identical to the hormones you naturally produce, has been intentionally orchestrated by the pharmaceutical companies. Why? Because they can't patent bioidentical hormones. By altering hormones, the drug companies create a non-natural, synthetic hormone that they can then patent and make millions of dollars from. They create a one-size-fits-all hormone patch or pill. Not only are the synthetic hormones themselves damaging, but the one-size-fits-all dose is dangerous on two levels: first, it doesn't require your doctor to have your hormone levels tested to see which hormones need replacing, and second, it may be either providing too much or too little of the missing hormone and/or the wrong hormones altogether!

Bioidentical hormones are only prescribed after taking a hormone test (a saliva test, not a blood test) and are specifically mixed by a compounding pharmacy to meet your individual hormonal needs. Bioidentical hormones are not one-size-fits-all. This tailoring makes taking bioidentical hormones safer than synthetic ones, but still does not remove the unknown risks associated with their long-term use. If your doctor does

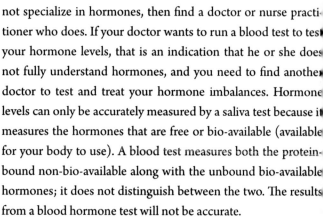

not specialize in hormones, then find a doctor or nurse practitioner who does. If your doctor wants to run a blood test to test your hormone levels, that is an indication that he or she does not fully understand hormones, and you need to find another doctor to test and treat your hormone imbalances. Hormone levels can only be accurately measured by a saliva test because it measures the hormones that are free or bio-available (available for your body to use). A blood test measures both the protein-bound non-bio-available along with the unbound bio-available hormones; it does not distinguish between the two. The results from a blood hormone test will not be accurate.

The difference between natural bioidentical hormones and synthetic hormones has been promoted by some as being like night and day; synthetics have been proven to cause breast cancer and bioidenticals may actually work to prevent breast cancer. On the other hand, the pharmaceutical industry is working overtime to convince you and your doctors that there is no difference between the two. Here's the difference. A natural or bioidentical hormone is one that matches exactly what your own body produces. The molecular structure is exactly the same. Synthetic hormones do not molecularly match those that your own body produces. They are different from the hormones your body naturally produces.

How are these hormones made? With the exception of the synthetic hormone Premarin (made from pregnant horse urine), both bioidentical and synthetic hormones start from the same source--wild yam or soybeans. A substance called diosgenin is extracted from the plants and then modified to create hormones. Your body cannot modify diosgenin so taking wild yam or soy supplements will not affect your hormone levels. Although the creation of both bioidentical and synthetic hormones starts out with this same substance, bioidentical hormones are made to exactly match those your body naturally produces. Because they match those found in nature (your body), they cannot be patented. Synthetic hormones take that same substance, and by altering a few molecules, they create hormones that do not match the ones your body naturally produces. Why do they do that? For only one reason: so they can be patented. If the hormone is different from the one found naturally in your body, the drug company can hold a patent on that altered hormone and make lots of money because now no other company can produce that altered hormone. Because bioidenticals cannot be patented, and therefore no huge profits stand to be made, no big studies are being done on the long-term effects of using bioidentical hormones.

Suzanne Somers has become the face for bioidentical hormones in this country. She has been unfairly painted as a crazy woman trying to find the fountain of youth. However, to many women she is a hero, bringing attention to bioidentical hormones and their health benefits. She is not alone. Many prominent doctors in the United States support what she is saying. In fact, she didn't dream up bioidentical hormones; she simply did extensive research when she started to encounter health problems (including breast cancer) and based on her research, decided they were a safe way to balance her hormones. Suzanne is also a proponent of homeopathy; she is using Iscador, a homeopathic herbal remedy used in Europe to treat breast cancer.

BALANCING HORMONES WITH HOMEOPATHY

Bioidentical hormones appear to be safe, but the bottom line is no one really knows for sure. Because of that uncertainty, I wanted a second opinion before I made my decision. My second opinion on treating my hormone imbalances was from a nurse practitioner working with a major hospital in my area. I didn't know what to think when she said she balanced women's hormones using homeopathy. She had many concerns over the use of bioidentical hormones and did not feel they were safe. I was not familiar with homeopathy, so I did some research.

Developed in the eighteenth century by a German doctor, Samuel Hahnemann, homeopathy is based on the concept that "like heals like." Giving the patient extremely small doses of the same substance that is causing the illness or imbalance, diluted many times in distilled water, causes the body to heal itself. This is exactly how many vaccines and allergy medicines work. This tiny amount of the healing substance (it can be plant, mineral, animal, or chemical) creates an electromagnetic pattern in the water. This pattern is recognized by your body and repeated exposures to this pattern will cause the body to heal itself. This

I strongly urge you to set aside whatever preconceived notions you have about Suzanne Somers and read her latest book, *Breakthrough*. In this book, she interviews many leading doctors. Their answers regarding diet, specific supplements, and hormones are nothing short of illuminating. Every woman I have suggested read this book has thanked me profusely.

is called resonance. Critics, like the American Cancer Society, say this is ridiculous. But, as it turns out, much of current scientific research on nanotechnology is based on the very same underlying principle of homeopathy—that the use of very small particles is very powerful. The United States government is pouring millions of dollars into research on nanotechnologies, not because they are "ridiculous," but because they work. Research into new cancer medicines is also focused on using nanotechnology.

Nanobees are an example of how nanotechnology may change the way cancer is treated in the future. A bee toxin called Melittin is attached to nanoparticles (structures smaller than 100 nanometers) that are engineered to travel directly to cancer cells. These nanobees use the toxin to destroy cancer cells while not harming healthy cells.

Homeopathy has a 200-year history and has a great deal of clinical evidence, including double-blind clinical trials in humans, that prove its effectiveness. In *The Homeopathic Revolution*, Dana Ullman says, "Homeopathic medicine is so widely practiced by physicians in Europe that it is no longer considered 'alternative medicine' there." He adds that "30% of French doctors and 20% of German doctors use homeopathic medicine regularly, while more than 40% of British physicians refer patients to homeopathic doctors and almost half of Dutch physicians consider homeopathic medicines to be effective."

Homeopathy came under fierce attack when in 1846, the American Medical Association was established, primarily to stop the growth of homeopaths in the United States. Homeopathic doctors had been criticizing standard medical practices of the time such as bloodletting and using toxic doses of mercury, antimony, arsenic, and lead (practices today recognized as barbaric), and more and more patients were going to homeopathic doctors because they were getting better results. Homeopaths also criticized the prescribing of multiple drugs because of the dangerous effects of their combinations. Because pharmacists (called apothecaries at the time) made much more money from the doctors who prescribed multiple drugs and in higher doses, the apothecaries also disliked homeopaths. But the main reason for the vilification of homeopathic doctors is that homeopathy represents a different form of medicine. Conventional (allopathic) medicine focuses on suppressing or controlling the symptoms of a disease or illness. Homeopathy believes that symptoms are the body's natural way of defending against a disease. Therefore, homeopathic medicines mirror the defense and aim to treat the underlying physiological and psychological causes of the disease, bringing the body back into balance. Unfortunately, this antagonistic relationship continues today.

If your doctor scoffs at the mention of homeopathy, consider this: the homeopathic principle of "like cures like" is used in choosing radiation to treat cancer; high doses of radiation cause cancer and low doses kill cancer. Other examples using this homeopathic principle are digitalis to treat heart conditions (digitalis causes heart conditions) and Ritalin given to hyperactive children (Ritalin is an amphetamine-like drug that causes hyperactivity).

Homeopathy works to uncover the causes of the hormonal imbalances and works to correct them, not just alleviate the symptoms. If you have hormone receptor positive breast cancer, or if you don't have breast cancer and want to prevent it, and you are rightly concerned about using bioidentical hormones to balance your hormones, you should make an appointment with a health care professional who practices homeopathy. These practitioners can be hard to find. Often they are called naturopathic doctors or nurse practitioners. One of the best places to find this type of medical practitioner in your area, especially if you live in a small town, is to visit a non-chain health store and talk to the staff. Make sure that you get a qualified practitioner with a certification and a degree.

Dr. Theresa Dale is the leading expert on balancing women's hormones using homeopathy. Her approach to balancing hormones is to work to bring the whole body back into balance so that your body will heal itself and in doing so, re-regulate all hormone levels. This method of hormonal balancing is not as fast or easy as taking a pill or applying a cream, but there is absolutely no risk of it causing breast cancer.

Because I have concerns about the long-term safety of using bioidentical hormones, I sought out a naturopathic doctor to work with in correcting my hormonal imbalances. She is a proponent of Dr. Dale's methods. I asked her if she would be willing to share her experiences in balancing women's hormones using

I strongly encourage you to read Dr. Theresa Dale's book, *Revitalize Your Hormones; Dr. Dale's 7 Steps to a Happier, Healthier and Sexier You.* You can also visit her Web site: www.wellnesscenter.net.

If you want more information on a homeopathic program for balancing your hormones, you may contact Celeste Hughes, ND, HHP, (doctor of naturopathy and Holistic Healthcare Practitioner) at (515) 225-4347 or by email at greatearthiowa@aol.com.

Here are some books and Web sites that can provide you with more information about homeopathy.

Books:

The Homeopathic Revolution by Dana Ullman, MPH

Homeopathy: Science or Myth by Bill Gray, MD

The Emerging Science of Homeopathy by Paolo Bellavite, MD, and Andrea Signorini, MD

Impossible Cure: The Promise of Homeopathy by Amy L. Lansky, PhD

Web sites:

www.homeopathyhome.com

www.homeopathic.com

www.wellnesscenter.net

HRT or BHRT (synthetic or bioidentical hormone replacement therapies) and homeopathy.

She told me that several years ago she started seeing women who had been on HRT and BHRT who had experienced good results initially, but after six months to a year, saw their initial symptoms return. Some women actually felt worse than before they had started the hormone therapies. She discovered that what these women were experiencing was a toxic buildup of these hormones in their bodies, from both the synthetic and bio-identical hormones. These toxic levels of hormones could eventually lead to hormone-sensitive cancers, such as breast cancer. Working in conjunction with a nurse practitioner who specializes in women's hormones, she started treating these women with a homeopathic approach that involved detoxifying their bodies, diet and lifestyle adjustments, and individualized homeopathic medicines. This approach yielded an over 80 percent improvement for these women. One woman was so thankful to finally have found a treatment that relieved all her symptoms and put her back on the road to good health she wrote, "Dear Celeste, I really didn't think I had any options left. I was overweight, had low blood sugar episodes, panic attacks, constipation, was under stress, and had endometriosis with abnormal Pap tests. I was tired of taking too many prescriptions. I was taking two, then four, then six. Enough was enough! I wanted an alternative but didn't know where to look. I can't tell you how great I feel now. I will always be grateful for the homeopathic program."

THE IODINE CONNECTION

It appears that iodine deficiency is also a factor in creating hormonal imbalance. As mentioned in Chapter Five, iodine deficiency has been linked to an increased risk for breast cancer. Among the three estrogens—estrone, estradiol, and estriol—an imbalance with and elevated level of estradiol is a major risk factor for breast cancer. Dr. David Brownstein, author of *Iodine: Why You Need It Why You Can't Live Without It*, discovered both in his practice and in research that an imbalance in these estrogens is promoted by a deficiency in iodine. A colleague of Dr. Brownstein's, Dr. Jonathan Wright also found that iodine supplementation helps to balance the three estrogens. Dr. Brownstein also notes that "iodine down-regulated [lowered] several estrogen responsive genes" and that it "could enhance the efficacy of Tamoxifen therapy."

These findings and much more information contained in Dr. Brownstein's book clearly indicate that iodine supplementation may be an important piece of the puzzle in creating and maintaining hormonal balance and preventing breast cancer.

MY LESSON IN HORMONAL IMBALANCE

I was astonished to learn that by the time you are able to feel a lump, or it is detectable on a mammogram, that cancer has most likely been growing for anywhere from five to ten years! Like other women diagnosed with breast cancer who have no family history of the disease (90 percent of all breast cancer is not inherited), I sought for a reason I got breast cancer. Was it something I did? Knowing that my small tumor had been growing for anywhere from five to ten years made me look back at my health and my lifestyle starting ten years ago. When I did that, I realized that I may have unknowingly caused my own breast cancer! Prior to being diagnosed with fibroid tumors, my diet contained a high intake of sugars and refined carbohydrates (the bad ones). Running a small business and working 24/7, I led a very stressful life, which I now know increased my cortisol levels (another breast cancer risk factor). I also realized that another untreated hormonal imbalance (estrogen dominance) that had caused my fibroid tumors was quite possibly to blame. I now wonder if I had known to seek treatment for my hormonal imbalances years ago when symptoms first appeared, and had known about the dietary factors that cause cancer and had changed my diet, would I have gotten breast cancer? I can't know for sure, but I don't want to take that chance again.

Several weeks after my mastectomy, I had my hormone levels checked with a saliva test. The results showed estrogen imbalances and a sky-high cortisol level. This may not be the smoking gun in regards to my breast cancer, but I am certain these imbalances played a part, and I am focused on getting my entire body and my hormones back into balance. I am working with a qualified health practitioner who specializes in hormonal balancing to do that. Hormones are a very tricky, delicate matter.

For more information on hormones, hormones testing, and information on the symptoms of hormonal imbalance, please consider checking out these books and Web sites.

Books:

Hormones Made Simple by John R. Lee, MD

The Wisdom of Menopause by Christiane Northrup, MD

What Your Doctor May Not Tell You About Breast Cancer by John R. Lee, MD

Web sites:

www.johnleemd.com. Select RESOURCES from the menu for the hormone balance tests.

www.virginiahopkinstestkits.com

www.wellnesscenter.net Hormone test kits also available through this Web site.

For this reason, I urge all women to work only with a health practitioner who specializes in hormone balancing. This will most likely not be your personal physician.

I also had my iodine levels tested through a 24-hour iodine loading test to check for low iodine levels. While my saliva hormone test showed normal levels of thyroid hormones T3 and T4 and TSH, the results of the 24–hour iodine-loading test indicated that I have a considerable iodine deficiency. I was put on 50 mg of Iodoral per day along with ATP Cofactors (B2 and B3 vitamins) that enhance the transport of iodine into cells and vital organs. My iodine deficiency may have been the underlying cause of my hormonal imbalances and my breast cancer.

GOOGLE SEARCH SUGGESTIONS

- Estrone
- Estradiol
- Estriol
- Progesterone
- Testosterone
- DHEA
- Pregnenolone
- Thyroid
- Melatonin
- Cortisol
- Dr. Joel Hargrove and bioidentical hormones
- Synthetic hormones and breast cancer
- Bioidentical hormone
- Bioidentical hormone use in Europe
- Bioidentical hormones versus synthetic hormones
- Are bioidentical hormones safe?
- Balancing hormones with homeopathy
- Iodine and hormone imbalance
- Dr. Brownstein and iodine

Note: in some instances the spelling is bio-identical. Hormone replacement therapy using bioidentical hormones is referred to as BHRT (not HRT).

When a well-packaged web of lies has been sold gradually to the masses over generations, the truth will seem utterly preposterous and its speaker a raving lunatic.

DRESDEN JAMES

Who Controls Your Cancer Treatment?

I feel I am about to tell you there is no Santa Claus.

When we were kids, we believed Santa Claus was a kindly old man from the North Pole who watched us all year to see if we were naughty or nice and would shower us with gifts on Christmas Day. As we grew up, we realized he was a myth, that Santa was really a man in the mall being paid to dress up and lie to us. That news came as a shock; we wanted so badly to believe the myth.

Today, drug companies, the National Cancer Institute, and the American Cancer Society are saying, "Ho! Ho! Ho!" all the way to the bank, and we are still children believing the myth that they are working to prevent and cure cancer. Like your parents who eventually had to tell you that there is no Santa Claus, I am not trying to be cruel. If you are going to avoid getting breast cancer or getting the wrong treatment for breast cancer, you must know the truth.

Who is really in control of the treatments you receive if you have breast cancer may shock you. Certain drugs and treatment protocols are recommended over others—not necessarily because they are better for patients, but because they may be more profitable for the drug companies that make them.

Dr. Linus Pauling, the only person ever to be awarded two unshared Nobel Prizes put it this way: "Everyone should know that the 'war on cancer' is largely a fraud."

The Truth About Drug Companies: How They Deceive Us and What to Do About It by Marcia Angell, MD, former editor of the prestigious *New England Journal of Medicine,* is one of the most enlightening books about this. *Publishers Weekly* says her book "presents a searing indictment of 'big pharma' as corrupt and corrupting: of Congress, through huge campaign contributions; of the FDA, which is funded in part by the very companies it oversees; and, perhaps most shocking, of members of the medical profession and its institutions. Angell delineates how the drug giants, such as Pfizer and AstraZeneca, pay physicians to prescribe their products with gifts, junkets, and marketing programs disguised as 'professional education.'"

One article, "Senate Hearing Details Influence of Drug Companies in Doctor Education," by John Fauber, published July of 2009 in the *Wisconsin Journal Sentinel* in a series of investigative reports on drug money influence at the University of Wisconsin School of Medicine, states, "Every dollar spent by a drug company on doctor education generated $3.56 in increased revenue." That's increased revenue for drug companies.

The complete *Wisconsin Journal Sentinel* article is available at www.jsonline.com/news/wisconsin/52008087.html.

The same article quotes Steven Nissen, chairman of cardiovascular medicine at The Cleveland Clinic, as saying, "CME [Continuing Medical Education] has largely evolved into marketing, cleverly disguised as education."

Drug representatives call on doctors for one purpose—to sell drugs. John Kopchinski, former Pfizer drug representative and whistle-blower in the most recent case against Pfizer, told Reuters news organization, "At Pfizer I was expected to increase profits at all costs, even when sales meant endangering lives." On September 2, 2009, news headlines revealed that Pfizer had just made its fourth settlement of the decade with the US government for charges of healthcare fraud. In this newest case, Pfizer must pay $2.3 million in penalties—the largest healthcare fraud settlement in the history of the US Justice Department—for marketing drugs to doctors for uses for which they have not been approved. According to a related *New York Times* article, Pfizer is now planning to move heavily into the cancer drug market.

When I started to research this topic, I thought I would have to do a lot of digging to uncover the truth about how drug companies influence your doctor's education. Because most women were not aware of it, I thought the evidence would be hard to find. I was wrong. The connections are so well-known that the medical establishment itself and prominent medical journals are outraged and calling for action. Entire books have been written on the subject. Articles in print and online abound.

Magazine articles on the topic, for example, include:

- *British Medical Journal*: "Doctors' Education: The Invisible Influence of Drug Company Sponsorship"
- *San Francisco Business Times*: "Pharmaceutical Company Gives New Meaning to 'Spin Doctors'"
- *New England Journal of Medicine*: "Doctors and Drug Companies"
- *New York Times*: "The Danger in Drug Kickbacks"

A small sampling of Web site articles on connections between drug companies, doctors, and the NCI, ACS, and the FDA includes:

- www.time.com/time/healtharticle/0,8599,1883449,00.html. "Is Drug Company Money Tainting Medical Education?"
- www.nybooks.com/articles/22237. "How Drug Companies Educate Doctors" by Dr. Marcia Angell, former head of the American Medical Association
- www.thedcasite.com/chemotherapy_kickbacks.html. "Chemotherapy Kickbacks"
- www.newswithviews.com/Richards/byron34.htm. "How the FDA is becoming a Drug Company"
- www.alkalizeforhealth.net/boycottACS.htm. "Boycott the ACS"
- www.preventcancer.com/losing/acs/tikkun_2000.htm. "High Stakes of Cancer Prevention"
- www.sierraclub.org/sierra/199909/cancer.asp. "Cancer, Inc."

To summarize the outrage, big drug companies now have a stranglehold on how doctors are educated, on how cancer research money is spent, on what treatments are prescribed, and on what effective treatments get covered up. The goal is no

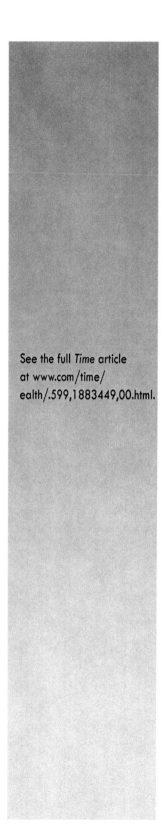

See the full *Time* article at www.com/time/ealth/.599,1883449,00.html.

longer finding a cure for cancer; it is to make profits for drug companies.

The influence that the large drug companies now have, beginning with your doctors' education, continuing throughout their practice, and influencing their treatment recommendations, has become so great that Congress, the American Medical Association (AMA), and the American Medical Student Association (AMSA) are all demanding that something be done to break these ties.

This year a group of medical students protested outside Harvard University calling for a severing of the ties between that university and the big pharmaceutical companies. According to an article, "Is Drug Company Money Tainting Medical Education?", published in *TIME* in March of this year: "Of Harvard's 8,900 professors and lecturers, 1,600 admit that either they, or a family member, have had some kind of business link to drug companies—sometimes worth hundreds of thousands of dollars—that could bias their teaching or research. . . . Additionally, pharma contributed more than $11.5 million to the school last year for research and continuing education classes."

Harvard Medical School is not alone. The same pattern is repeated in many medical schools throughout the country. Besides giving outright donations of millions of dollars to institutions for research and education, drug companies sponsor medical "education" seminars that count as fulfilling a doctor's continuing education requirements. The problem is this "education" is actually marketing: promoting a newer drug or medical device. New isn't always better, but it is almost always more profitable.

The situation is so serious that the March *TIME* article cited above declared, "Federal officials revealed a newly aggressive plan to begin pursuing civil and criminal charges against doctors who accept kickbacks or demand speaking or consulting fees for prescribing drugs or medical devices." Many doctors are concerned also. PharmedOut is an organization set up to help doctors resist drug promotions that are inappropriate.

According to Dr. Samuel S. Epstein, professor of occupational and environmental medicine at the University of Illinois School of Public Health, drug company influence goes beyond medical education. It extends also to the US Food and Drug

Administration (FDA) and major cancer organizations. The boards of the National Cancer Institute (NCI), the American Cancer Society (ACS), and the FDA are filled with representatives from the companies that make cancer treatment drugs. The board of the American Cancer Society Foundation (the fundraising group of the ACS) includes David Bethune, president of the huge drug company Lederle Laboratories. Bethune is also the vice-president of American Cyanamid, a company that manufactures chemical fertilizers and herbicides.

That's just the tip of the iceberg. In their book, *The High Stakes of Cancer Prevention*, Samuel Epstein and Liza Gross document how these cancer organizations also have actually worked to block legislation aimed at cancer prevention. For example, in 1992 a scientific advisory group called the International Joint Commission (IJC) proposed a global phaseout of specific organochloride pesticides found to cause breast cancer (when the government of Israel banned these pesticides, breast cancer rates dropped there by 8 percent). The American Cancer Society sided with the Chlorine Institute and opposed the ban. In 1977 and 1978 the ACS opposed regulations for hair dyes that were shown to cause breast cancer in rats. You can read many more examples in Dr. Epstein's book.

A book devoted solely to exposing the link between the FDA and the pharmaceutical industry is *Fight For Your Health: Exposing the FDA's Betrayal of America*, by Byron J. Richards. This book exposes the conflict of interest that now exists in the FDA due to its being headed and controlled by individuals with ties to the pharmaceutical industry. Richards says, "The priority of these men is to rush unproven drugs to market, for the financial benefit of Wall Street and Big Pharma." Richards also says about the FDA, "They are actively working to suppress natural-health options which hold tremendous health-care potential."

According to an article at www.projectcensored.org, the ACS spends only one quarter of its budget on research, but 60 percent on salaries and bonuses, and it holds millions of dollars in reserves. It quotes the conclusion of *The Chronicle of Philanthropy* (www.philanthropy.com) that "The ACS is more interested in accumulating wealth than saving lives."

Women turn to these two big cancer organizations for all their information on treatments, not knowing the biases of the

I recommend you visit www.projectcensored.org and read the article, "Financially Bloated American Cancer Society Fails To Prevent Cancer." Use the site's search function to look for American Cancer Society.

If you want to read some enlightening criticism of the ACS from leading doctors, researchers, and former NCI representatives, go to www.encognitive.com/node/1212.

Books about the drug industry:

Money Driven Medicine by Maggie Mahar

Our Daily Meds by Melody Petersen

The High Stakes of Cancer Prevention by Samuel S. Epstein, MD, and Liza Gross

The Politics of Cancer by Samuel S. Epstein, MD

Reclaiming Our Health by John Robbins

Patient No More: The Politics of Breast Cancer by Sharon Blatt

The Truth About The Drug Companies: How They Deceive Us and What to Do About It by Marcia Angell, MD

When Healing Becomes a Crime by Kenny Ausubel

The Cancer Industry by Ralph Moss, PhD

Fighting for Your Health: Exposing the FDA's Betrayal of America by Byron J. Richards, CCN

information they receive. All the articles referenced here and the books I list in the sidebar provide more evidence of how these organizations appear to be primarily interested in promoting the welfare and profits of the drug companies.

BREAST CANCER AWARENESS MONTH

Breast Cancer Awareness Month was created in 1985 by drug company Zeneca. At that time Zeneca was owned by Imperial Chemical Industries, which produces pesticides, paper, and plastics. Imperial Chemicals was sued in 1990 for dumping DDT and PCBs (both cancer-causing chemicals linked to breast cancer) into Los Angeles and Long Beach harbors. Zeneca acquired a chain of cancer treatment centers in 1997 just before merging with Astra, now becoming AstraZeneca, the world's third largest drug company.

According to Dr. Samuel Epstein, "You've got a company that's a spin-off of one of the world's biggest manufacturers of carcinogenic chemicals, they've got control of breast cancer treatment, they've got control of chemoprevention studies, and now they have control of cancer treatment in eleven centers—which are clearly going to be prescribing the drugs they manufacture."

AstraZeneca controls all literature associated with Breast Cancer Awareness Month, and the literature focuses on mammograms. Not one word or one dime devoted to prevention. Do you really think AstraZeneca wants to prevent breast cancer when there is so much money to be made on the treatments?

PROFIT, NOT PREVENTION, IS THE GOAL

In my research, I found a fascinating report by a leading market research firm that provides revenue forecasts for drug companies for 2000-2010.

The following excerpts are chilling:

- "With increasing public awareness about breast cancer and its treatments, the market for breast cancer therapies is primed for expansion."
- "These sectors [I assume they meant current breast cancer therapies] also face a threat from emerging therapies that promise to improve the quality of the patient's life."

- "In order to counter the effects of this loss, large pharmaceutical companies need to fill their pipelines with newly patented therapies and transition patients onto the next generation therapies."

"U.S. Breast Cancer Therapeutics Markets" was produced by Research and Markets, one of the world's largest market research firms. To read the full report from which these citations are taken, go to the Web site listed in the sidebar on this page.

Does this sound as if there is any concern for women with breast cancer getting the best treatment? It's about profits and market shares and patenting new drugs that may or may not be effective but that generate more dollars. And how do the pharmaceutical companies push these new drugs? By marketing to doctors via "educational seminars" at expensive resorts, expensive lunches, with gifts, bonuses, or kickbacks—or by simply providing the doctor with biased reports on the efficacy of a new, and more expensive, drug.

When women understand this dynamic for who controls cancer treatments, they can be on guard, ask questions, and do research to get the best treatment for themselves, not just the most profitable one for others.

GOOGLE SEARCH SUGGESTIONS:

- The influence of drug companies on doctors
- The influence of drug companies on medicine
- Chemotherapy kickbacks
- Who heads the FDA?
- Board members of the American Cancer Society
- Board members of the National Cancer Institute

Here is the Web site with the full text of the report from Research and Markets: www.researchandmarkets.com/reports/594400/u_s_breast_cancer_theraputics_markets.htm.

Here is another interesting Web site: www.bcaction.org.

We doctors need you to help us think better. We need you to question us and engage us from a position of knowledge about how and when we think well and how and when we go astray.... It's really hard to be a doctor. But it's much harder to be a patient.

DR. JEROME GROOPMAN

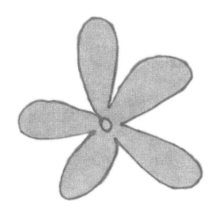

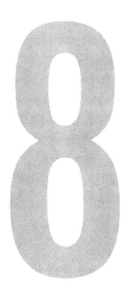

Help Your Doctor Heal You

When women fail to do their own research, it is usually because they choose to rely on their doctors as their sole source of breast cancer information. They see no need to research on their own. Once they understand how cancer starts, how it can be prevented, how a strong immune system can kill cancer cells naturally, and how the drug companies control cancer treatment, they see the need to do their own research about their specific form of cancer. They start to ask their doctors questions about their breast cancer treatment.

Most doctors are caring, competent people who truly want to help patients. However, doctors are only human, and they think in the same fallible way that all humans do. Understanding and recognizing their patterns of thought will help you to see reasons doctors can make mistakes and why it is your job to help them avoid those mistakes.

In the *New York Times* best seller, *How Doctors Think*, Jerome Groopman, MD, a chair of medicine at Harvard Medical School, states, "Experts studying misguided care have recently concluded that the majority of [medical] errors are due to flaws in physician thinking, not technical mistakes." He goes on to state that based on other studies, approximately 15 percent of all diagnoses are wrong. In other words, it's not that someone switched a patient's

For more information, read the book *How Doctors Think* by Jerome Groopman, MD.

X-rays or read the wrong lab test, the problem lies in how doctors think. So, it is critical to understand how doctors think so we are not afraid to do our own research and ask questions.

Dr. Groopman discovered that a patient's questions disrupt a doctor's thinking pattern, resulting in the patient receiving better care. Because I want you to be that patient, I'll walk through some of these dangerous thinking patterns with you. Although listed separately, most of these patterns of thinking are at work simultaneously and can lead to a cascade of little mistakes in treatment or to one major error.

PATTERN RECOGNITION

Doctors are trained to evaluate patient symptoms and render a diagnosis for which they prescribe treatment, if needed. If a patient has symptoms A, B, and C, but not E, the patient's diagnosis is X. If the patient had symptom E, the diagnosis would be Y. For diagnosis X, the doctor knows to prescribe treatment X. This method of determining diagnosis and treatment is so standard, that there are computer programs based on pattern recognition. These programs are called medical templates.

I witnessed my oncologist using a template when, during my initial visit, he went to a site at www.adjuvant.com, entered data from my pathology report, and printed out a chemotherapy recommendation for me. What's wrong with that? It works if you are a typical patient with typical symptoms, typical physical history, or typical pathology. But defining typical is very difficult. Many women are not typical, and many cancers are not typical either. By using pattern recognition, with or without the medical template program, your doctor will most likely miss everything about you and your cancer that is not typical. If you don't ask questions, or bring to light something in your pathology report, medical history, or lifestyle that might make you atypical, you risk getting the wrong diagnosis and treatment.

In the average 15-minute office visit, a doctor does not have time to ask a lot of questions to determine who is typical and who is not. In a fascinating book, *Every Patient Tells a Story: How and Why Doctors Misdiagnose*, Dr. Lisa Sanders' studies reveal that on average, a doctor gives a patient only twenty seconds to talk. One physician in Dr. Groopman's book likened the hectic schedules of most doctors to a fast-moving train with a patient in each window. Unless something happens to slow down that train (such as your asking questions), each patient is like a face in the train window—just a blur.

Personally, I think that pattern recognition is a dangerous mode of thinking that leads to most inappropriate or unnecessary treatments for breast cancer. And all standard treatments for breast cancer have serious consequences. Any mistakes made that result in unnecessary surgery, radiation, chemotherapy, or toxic drugs will be life-changing for the patient.

My treatment experience showed me the need to ask questions to slow down my fast-moving train and become more than a blur. My doctors didn't think that the tiny lump in my breast was cancer, so they removed just the lump itself and sent it in for a biopsy. No surrounding tissue was removed; in other words, I did not have a lumpectomy. As soon as the pathology report came back indicating ductal carcinoma in situ (a pre-cancerous condition referred to as DCIS), I was sent to an oncologist. The oncologist said he would schedule me for radiation treatments.

I had already done research on treatment for DCIS and learned that radiation is not warranted if a patient is at low risk for invasive cancer. Risk is determined by several factors in the pathology report from a lumpectomy. In my research, I had also learned there was a good chance that the radiation itself could cause my non-life-threatening pre-cancerous condition to become life-threatening invasive cancer.

When I raised these questions, my first oncologist was not willing to answer them or discuss them with me. I refused radiation treatment and looked for another doctor. I scheduled an appointment with a specialist at a breast cancer center. He listened to my objections to radiation, went over my pathology report with me, and agreed that I needed a lumpectomy in order to determine my risk.

He sent me to talk to a radiation specialist who also was willing to discuss all the studies I brought with me, and he also agreed that I needed the lumpectomy. He also concurred that if pathology results showed that I was at low risk for recurrence, there was mounting evidence indicating that radiation might not be needed or beneficial.

By doing research and asking questions, I slowed the train down and was seen as a person instead of a blur.

REPRESENTATIVENESS ERRORS

From time to time we all make representativeness errors in thinking. Medical representativeness errors occur when a doctor's thinking is guided by a prototype, such as, "She looks healthy so it can't be anything serious."

A representativeness error may have impacted my initial treatment. I am trim and active and am told I look younger than my calendar age. In other words, I look healthy. When I went to see my family doctor after discovering a small, hard lump in my left breast, she said she thought it was probably nothing and that we could just watch it for a while. I wanted it out! The surgeon who removed it said he was sure it was just a calcification. If I were overweight, appeared unhealthy, and looked older than my calendar age, would my doctors have been as reassuring? If it's simply a matter of reassuring a patient, that's not a big issue. But if a patient appears healthy and therefore a serious diagnosis is automatically dismissed as a possibility, certain symptoms also may be dismissed or overlooked—leading to an error in diagnosis. According to Dr. Groopman's research, this is not just speculation, it happens often.

LOOKING FOR THE ZEBRA

In medical school, doctors are taught: "If you hear galloping, look for a horse not a zebra." In other words, look for the most obvious answer or diagnosis, not the rare one. But, what if you are the patient with the rare disease? Although this thinking is great to help doctors avoid ordering unnecessary tests, it is dangerous if your breast cancer is a zebra. Therefore, a patient needs to know and understand her breast cancer pathology in order to ask those questions that will make her doctor pay attention to the individuality of her breast cancer. This is especially true with the form of breast cancer I had: triple negative. This type of breast cancer is poorly understood, so it is often a zebra.

CONFORMITY

Conformity thinking could be named peer pressure. Peer pressure is not just the territory of adolescence; it is the *modus operandi* in medicine. If a doctor writes an article, it must be peer-reviewed to have any credibility. The establishment of standard of care is based on consensus, not necessarily on sound studies. Once a standard of care is established, all doctors are supposed to follow that practice and are disparaged if they deviate from it. In extreme cases, they may lose their license. As a patient, you will most likely win a lawsuit against a doctor if he deviated from that standard of care. Where is the incentive for doctors to do research on their own? There simply is none. Where is the incentive for a doctor to discuss or offer an alternative treatment? There isn't any. You, the patient, will have to lead your doctor to think outside the box.

UNCERTAINTY

Medicine is a field of uncertainty, based only on current knowledge. And current knowledge is always limited because it does not include what is yet to be discovered. But we, the patients, don't view it that way. We look to our doctors for all the answers. We expect them to know everything when they don't and simply can't.

Thousands of years ago everyone was certain the earth was flat. They were certain because no one had yet discovered or proved it was round. The earth didn't suddenly change its shape. It had always been round but no one knew that until being taught differently. At first that knowledge was speculative, based on observing the planets. But when Ferdinand Magellan sailed *around* the world, it was proven. Cancer doctors believe what they have been taught. Their training is almost always limited to radiation, pharmaceuticals, and surgery. Unless they take it upon themselves to investigate beyond the limits of those treatments, they will never know about other treatments that may be as effective, or more effective, and less toxic to the rest of the body. Many cancer doctors have gone beyond what they have been taught. They are the resources I have used.

Dr. David Servan-Schreiber was certain that the standard cancer treatments would eradicate his brain cancer. But when the tumor came back, he set out to find a better and more effective way to treat cancer. His book, *Anti-Cancer: A New Way of Life*, documents his findings.

LIABILITY

Because patients view their doctors as superhuman and unable to make mistakes, they are quick to sue if they feel their doctor made a mistake. Although some doctors deserve to be sued, they are the exception. But the fear of being sued is very real. Although doctors may know the alternative care information found in this book, they may be reluctant to offer anything other than the accepted standard of care for fear of being sued.

So, although your doctor may not prescribe supplements or hormonal balancing for fear of opening himself up to liability, you can and should inform your doctor of any "non-standard" methods you are using. You will often find that although they cannot approve your choices, they are willing to work with you.

Doctors care about their patients. But doctors are human. They have been trained to think in specific ways and to select specific treatments that may not always be best for individual patients. Doing your own research and then asking your doctor educated questions can create a partnership that will help to treat your breast cancer in the most appropriate way.

We treat a large number of women with chemotherapy to help the ones who will actually benefit from it.

ROBERT C. BAST, JR., MD
VICE PRESIDENT FOR TRANSITIONAL RESEARCH
M.D. ANDERSON CANCER CENTER

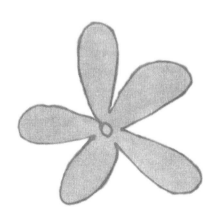

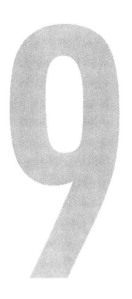

Chemotherapy: A Near-Death Experience

When my mother told me, "Don't run with scissors," or "Don't play in the street," I pressed her for a reason. If I understood the reason why my actions might hurt me or someone else, I would obey my mother. If her reasons didn't make sense or were just arbitrary ("because I said so," for example), I disobeyed the rule and did as I pleased. My poor mother!

Although my relentless need to know and fully understand made my mother's life difficult, it has served me well. I don't simply take someone's word. If something doesn't seem logical or make sense, I dig for the truth. And I delve into any subject that interests me: politics, science, art, religions, anthropology, history—and now breast cancer.

Once diagnosed with breast cancer I questioned every test, procedure, report, and treatment proposed. Nobody was going to do anything to my body unless I understood what was being done and why. No one mentioned the word chemotherapy to me when I was first diagnosed, but when I hear the word "cancer" my mind leaps to "chemotherapy." After all, that's the picture we all have of a cancer patient: bald and emaciated from chemotherapy treatments. So I immediately started my research on chemotherapy because I knew at some point a doctor was going to tell me I needed chemotherapy—and I was right.

You can read about this survey and many other responses from physicians regarding the effectiveness of chemotherapy at www. articlebase.com/cancer -articles/the-truth -about-chemotherapy-it-is -dangerous-906032.html.

Here's a book to consider for further reading: *Cancer: Why We Are Still Dying to Know the Truth* by Philip Day.

Before my cancer diagnosis, I had heard an interview on National Public Radio of a famous cancer specialist. I hadn't paid close attention, but the interviewer's final question made me stop and listen. She asked the doctor, "If you or a family member were diagnosed with cancer, would you undergo chemotherapy treatments?" After a long pause, he answered with a single word: "No."

At The McGill Cancer Center in Montreal, one of the most prestigious cancer centers in the world, 118 doctors were asked in a survey, if they or a family member were diagnosed with the specific type of cancer they were treating, would they undergo the chemotherapy regime they prescribed for their patients? Of the 79 doctors who answered the survey, 58 said no, that the chemotherapy drugs don't work and are toxic to the body's system. Yet these are the very doctors who routinely order chemotherapy for their patients.

Chemotherapy is poison. It is not a cure for breast cancer. It causes permanent damage to healthy cells. Chemotherapy drugs can themselves cause cancer. These are statements not usually made by oncologists. But they are true, and in order to decide whether or not to undergo chemotherapy treatments, you need to know the truth.

Oncologists are telling the truth when they say that chemotherapy has been shown to be "effective" against breast cancer or that certain breast cancers "respond" well to specific chemotherapy drugs. They are also telling the truth when they cite figures giving you a "percentage" of risk reduction of recurrence from chemotherapy. They never, however, talk about chemotherapy being a "cure" for breast cancer, because they know it is not.

So if these statements are true, and based on them it certainly sounds as if chemotherapy offers you a better chance of not having your cancer return, why would you not follow their advice? If chemotherapy itself were not life threatening, I would agree—what do you have to lose? But there is a lot to lose by undergoing chemotherapy and, it appears, little to gain.

DOES CHEMOTHERAPY WORK?

It's important to understand the terms that oncologists use when discussing the benefits of chemotherapy.

- **Effective:** Chemotherapy has been shown to be "effective" in treating breast cancer.

The FDA (the government organization that approves all chemotherapy drugs) defines a chemotherapy drug as being "effective" if it achieves a 50 percent or greater reduction in tumor size for twenty-eight days. You can die of breast cancer three months later, and that chemotherapy treatment is still considered to have been "effective." There is little, if any, correlation between shrinking a tumor for twenty-eight days and "curing" your breast cancer or even of prolonging your life.

- **Respond:** Breast cancer has been shown to "respond" well to chemotherapy.

  The meaning of the word "respond" is similar to the meaning of the word "effective." It merely means that in studies, some type of effect, either shrinking or slowed growth, has been demonstrated. But that effect can be for just a few days and be minimal.

- **Percentage risk:** Chemotherapy has been shown to lower the "percentage" of risk of recurrence.

  In *Calculated Risk*, Gerd Gigerenzer shows how data can be presented in such a way as to be true, but misleading. For example, if you were told that chemotherapy would reduce your risk of a recurrence of breast cancer by 25 percent, you'd probably be more inclined to undergo chemotherapy, even knowing the side effects and complications. But if you were told that out of 2,000 women, where 1,000 received chemotherapy and 1,000 did not, three women in the chemotherapy group had a recurrence and four women in the non-chemotherapy group had a recurrence, you might look at that and say, "That's not a substantial enough difference for me to accept the risks associated with chemotherapy."

Here's the problem. The 25 percent figure for reduction in breast cancer recurrence is one way of presenting the three versus four women in that study of the 2,000 women. How can that be? The percentage difference between the numbers three and four is 25 percent. It's still true, but certainly misleading and will lead you to make a very different decision.

If drug company representatives are trying to convince a doctor to order more chemotherapy treatments, you can be sure they are going to use that misleading, but true 25 percent figure in the educational materials given to oncologists. Unfortunately, your oncologist may then only present you with that misleading figure.

Another area of data manipulation is in the area of earlier detection. Due to the earlier detection of many breast cancers, which results in earlier treatment, statistics inaccurately attribute the longer life of the cancer patients to the treatments, when in fact it was due to earlier detection. This is especially true in the case of DCIS.

SURVIVAL RATES

The "survival rate" (also referred to as the overall survival rate) is the number to know. In the end, it doesn't matter if a tumor will shrink or cancer will show some "change" due to the chemotherapy drugs. The important information is how chemo-therapy will affect your survival rate. In other words, how much longer have women lived who underwent chemotherapy versus those who did not? These numbers are usually given in periods of years such as in 5-, 10-, 15-, and 20-year survival rates. Because many types of breast cancer typically don't recur for 10-15 years, you really need to know the longer term survival rates. According to my oncologist, it is now believed that one type of breast cancer called "triple negative," typically recurs in five years, sooner than most other types of breast cancer. Once you have been given that critical information, then you can decide if the negative side effects and possible complications from the chemotherapy treatments are worth the possibility of extending your life for whatever that given period of time is.

But be careful: as indicated above, these numbers can be deceiving. So, here are the questions you want answered: Are the survival rates quoted for the specific chemotherapy regimen (cocktail) you will receive, and for your specific type of breast cancer? The answer to those questions must be yes. The most important questions after that are: In the study from which the survival rate is being quoted, how many women were studied, how many received chemotherapy and how many did not, and how many women had the longer survival rates and how many did not, (not the percentage, you want the actual numbers), and what was the difference in the survival rates of these two groups of women (months? years?). You may have to ask your doctor for a copy of the study he is referencing to get all that information. Only when you have that exact information can you make an informed decision. You should also research other studies on your own as study results can vary a great deal and some "studies" are merely statistical predictions, not actual results.

In a study of one of the most common chemotherapy regimens given for postmenopausal, estrogen receptor-positive women (the largest group of women with breast cancer), researchers concluded that for the women treated with that chemotherapy regimen, "no significant survival benefit was observed."

LOCAL RECURRENCE AND RECURRENCE RATES

Local recurrence is a term that means cancer has returned to the original site—the breast. Local recurrence does not cause a woman to die from breast cancer. Only metastasis (distant recurrence) can lead to death. If your cancer stayed in your breast, it would be no problem. Many treatments offer only a reduced risk of local recurrence.

Distant recurrence or metastasis is what all women with breast cancer want to avoid. When prescribing a chemotherapy regimen, the rates of recurrence will also be quoted. You need to know if these rates refer only to local recurrence or recurrence to any site in the body. You want to ask those same important questions about the actual number of women (not the percentages) as cited above for survival rates. You also want to research other studies on your own.

When an oncologist says, "At present, we really don't have anything else to offer for treatment of breast cancer," that statement is true in the oncologist's mind. Chemotherapy has never been tested against a nutritional program to see which is more effective in fighting breast cancer. In other words, no large-scale study has been done to determine if boosting your own immune system would be a better and more effective way of preventing a recurrence or metastases than chemotherapy, which destroys your immune system. Given that all studies have to be funded and the vast majority are funded in some way by pharmaceutical companies, there is no incentive to conduct a study that might

Here's a book that may help you think this through: Questioning Chemotherapy by Dr. Ralph Moss.

Here is the source for the adjacent study: Hartman A.R., Fleming G.F., Dillon J.J., "Metaanalysis of Adjuvant cyclophosphamide/ methotrexate/5-fluorouracil Chemotherapy in Postmenopausal Women with Estrogen Receptor-Positive, Node Positive Breast Cancer," *Clinical Breast Cancer* 2001; 2(2):138-143. Study available at www.ncbi.nlm. nih.gov/pubmed/11899785.

determine that a specific nutritional program was more effective than chemotherapy.

Since oncologists receive a steady dose of "educational" materials from drug companies with misleading statistics on the benefits of chemotherapy, have seen no studies comparing the effectiveness of specific nutritional programs that boost your immune system (instead of destroying it), and have had little training in nutritional biochemistry, they truly do have nothing else to offer you than chemotherapy.

"EFFECTIVE" RE-EVALUATED

Shrinking a tumor for twenty-eight days—the FDA and drug companies criterion for effectiveness of a chemotherapy drug—is not my definition of effective. My definition of effective is the same as that of Webster and Oxford: "having a definite or desired effect." A twenty-eight day shrinkage is not my desired effect! A twenty-eight day shrinkage is ineffective.

Perhaps chemotherapy is, in fact, ineffective in treating breast cancer.

"Ineffective" is the conclusion of many noted scientists and doctors who have been working in the cancer field for decades. Dr. Ralph Moss has published an extensive study on the ineffectiveness of chemotherapy on all but a few cancers. Breast cancer is not one of the few. He says that the vast majority of cancers, including breast, colon, and lung cancers are barely touched by chemotherapy.

Dr. Ulrich Abel, a highly respected epidemiologist at Heidelberg Mannheim Tumor Clinic in Germany, crunched the numbers using data and statistics on chemotherapy from leading journals and thousands of studies from throughout the world to determine if chemotherapy was really working. His conclusion was that there was no scientific evidence that chemotherapy prolongs the life of patients.

CHEMOTHERAPY: WHAT IT IS AND HOW IT WORKS

Chemotherapy is based on the use of toxic, cell-damaging chemicals. It owes its origins to the mustard gas used during World War II. Asked by the US Department of Defense to

Here is a Web site to visit if you are considering chemotherapy: www.mercola.com/article/cancer/cancer_options.htm.

The Web site with Dr. Abel's findings is at www.encognitive.com/node/4361. It includes an in-depth, but understandable, account of his findings.

develop an alternative use for chemical warfare agents, two scientists discovered some of the anti-cancer activities of these toxic chemicals. Chemotherapy was first used to treat cancer in the 1940s, and its history as treatment for breast cancer is full of false hopes, overdoses, limited success, reassessment, corruption, and profit. In spite of this checkered history, today chemotherapy, drugs, and radiation are considered the only non-surgical treatments for breast cancer.

In my survey, many women viewed chemotherapy as the treatment they were most afraid of. As women, we are innately intuitive. It turns out that this is the treatment most to be feared, and therefore the one requiring most personal research.

Chemotherapy administers toxic drugs, either alone or in combinations called cocktails that are designed to kill your cancer cells faster than they kill your healthy cells. The theory is that because cancer cells are dividing rapidly, they will be killed first, before your healthy cells, which tend to divide more slowly. The problem is that your body is full of healthy cells that also divide rapidly. Those cells are found in your mouth, your hair, your digestive tract, your immune system, and in your brain. So, those cells are also killed right along with the cancer cells. Killing these non-cancerous cells is the reason for the side effects and complications listed below.

The goal is that your cancer dies from the chemotherapy drugs before the rest of your cells die. In many cases, you are brought as near death as possible in hopes of killing the cancer before you die. Many of those healthy cells that survive now have damaged DNA (a damage that can cause cancer). So, even if the chemotherapy kills your cancer cells (it never kills 100 percent of the cancer cells), you are left with a weakened immune system (a system you need to fight cancer cells) and cells with damaged DNA that can become cancer cells. The recurrence of cancer after chemotherapy may be a new cancer created by the chemotherapy itself.

Some chemotherapy drugs are more toxic than others, and used in combinations, they become more toxic still. As mentioned in Chapter Four, the presence in cancer cells of Nuclear Factor-KappaB (NF-KappaB) makes many cancer cells immune to the chemotherapy drugs. It has now been shown that chemotherapy drugs will actually cause an increase in

the production of NF-KappaB, which may lead to making any surviving cancer cells nearly impossible to kill.

CHEMOTHERAPY COMBINATIONS

If you are considering chemotherapy, ask your oncologist what drug "cocktail" he will be using for your treatments. Then research these drugs. Information is easily obtained on the Internet. When I did this research I learned that the National Cancer Institute now considers a group of chemicals called Taxanes (Taxol is the most common) proposed for my chemotherapy cocktail as being ineffective against the form of breast cancer I have.

Chemotherapy regimens are described like this: CAF, FAC, CEF, AC, or some other combination of letters. These letters stand for specific drugs. For example, CAF stands for the drug cocktail containing Cyclophosphamide, Doxorubicin (Adriamycin), and 5-fluorouracil. You can look each of those drugs up separately on the Internet.

SIDE EFFECTS VERSUS COMPLICATIONS

All chemotherapy drugs have both side effects and complications. Side effects are those adverse reactions that are known to happen. Complications are those adverse reactions that don't always happen, but have a certain percentage of risk of happening. You need to know the percentage of risk for complications from the chemotherapy drugs. The side effects are bad enough, but the complications are life threatening. What is the point of undergoing chemotherapy treatments in hopes of stopping your breast cancer from metastasizing, if in the process you end up with leukemia or permanent heart damage? By the way, women who die from the complications associated with chemotherapy are still considered a "success" story in the statistics and studies on chemotherapy. In other words, the treatment was a success, but the patient died.

Heart damage is one of the most serious and common complications from both chemotherapy and radiation treatments. Many women are not warned about this and do not realize that their long-term fatigue following these treatments may in fact be a result of damage to their heart muscle. This risk should be fully understood before undergoing treatment. Many doctors are now questioning the use of specific chemotherapy drugs used for breast cancer because of their high risk of heart damage.

COMMON SIDE EFFECTS AND COMPLICATIONS

Side effects of chemotherapy

- Fatigue
- Infertility
- Premature menopause
- Nausea and vomiting
- Hair loss
- Mouth and throat sores
- Risk of infections
- Anemia
- Immune suppressions
- Impaired memory
- Yeast infections
- Food aversions
- Abnormal bleeding
- Digestive problems
- Some degree of neurological (brain) damage
- Malnutrition
- Diarrhea
- Myeloid leukemia

Complications

- Liver damage
- Cardiac (heart) toxicity (especially with Doxorubicin, Adriamycin, Taxol and Taxotere—all commonly used for breast cancer chemo)
- Lung damage (combining chemo and radiation increases this risk)
- A secondary cancer
- Leukemia

TAMOXIFEN AND HERCEPTIN

Tamoxifen and Herceptin are considered endocrine therapy. Tamoxifen is used for women who are ER positive (estrogen receptor positive). It works by blocking the binding

In an article available at www.ahrp.org/cms/index2. php?option=comcontent&do pdf=1&id=328, this issue of long-term toxicity is clearly raised. This article states, "The survival benefit of a few percentage points estimated by these studies [clinical trials] may be offset by acute, chronic and late-onset toxicities."

You can read an interesting article relating to this at www.msnbc.msn.com/ id/21194.

of estrogen (estradiol) to estrogen receptors in breast tissue. It does, however, have side effects. Tamoxifen can increase a woman's risk for uterine cancer, dementia, and depression. It should not be taken for more than five years because it will start to have a reverse effect on breast tissue.

Herceptin is a drug given to women who are HER2-positive (HER-2 is a growth-promoting protein). It also has side effects. Herceptin is associated with serious heart muscle injury. Any woman on Herceptin should be monitored closely.

All of the risks and side effects of chemotherapy drugs can be easily found on the Internet.

MY CHEMOTHERAPY DECISION

I thought I was "cured" by having a double mastectomy. After all, I had no lymph node involvement, and my tumors were very small. But I discovered that because I had triple negative breast cancer, even though I had no lymph node involvement, I still had some risk of recurrence. So, after my double mastectomy I went to see my oncologist. I simply wanted to know if there were any tests I should have to detect if my cancer came back, since mammograms were no longer an option. I was shocked that my oncologist wanted to talk to me about chemotherapy.

Of course, I decided to do research to weigh the risks and benefits.

My research (much of which I have shared in this chapter) proved to me that the risks truly outweighed any small chance of a benefit. I also learned that the chemotherapy is now being questioned for women whose tumors are small and have no lymph node involvement. With all I now know about prevention, and ways to boost my immune system, I feel these offer just as good, if not a better way to prevent a recurrence, without any toxic side effects. It simply makes no sense to me to poison my entire body to rid myself of a few potential cancer cells when I know that my body makes and destroys cancer cells all the time. I also value my quality of life. Personally, I would rather die six months earlier than to live an extra six months sick from treatments. That is my personal decision; your decision may be a different one.

Ultimately the decision about chemotherapy belongs to you, the patient. Because the drugs are so extremely toxic, with

See these Web sites for more information about cancer therapies:

www.oncologySTAT.com

www.adjuvantonline.com

www.medlineplus.com

long-term side effects, it is important to weigh all the risks and benefits before making your decision. Only by doing your own research in this area will you discover if a specific chemotherapy drug has been recently called into question, or if a new long- or short-term toxicity has been detected. The field of oncology is continually in flux. New studies, warnings, and discoveries are made every day. Treatment recommendations are continually being questioned and reassessed. Your oncologist may not be aware of emerging treatment recommendations.

In *The 10 Best Questions for Surviving Breast Cancer*, Dede Bonner recommends asking your oncologist what is the most recent fact he or she has learned about breast cancer. If the oncologist is constantly learning about current studies, he or she will be able to answer almost immediately. If it takes a while to hear an answer, or if none is forthcoming, find another doctor.

Even if your doctor is up on current studies, getting a second opinion is important for all major medical decisions. It is especially important when it comes to any type of treatment for breast cancer. My advice is to find a doctor for a second opinion on your own. If you ask your doctor for a referral for a second opinion, you will most likely be sent to a doctor who shares your doctor's treatment biases. You want an independent second opinion. In the end, you may decide to have chemotherapy. You may decide not to. Whatever your decision, it is important that it be based on accurate information.

GOOGLE SEARCH SUGGESTIONS

- Survival rates for breast cancer
- Recurrence rates for breast cancer
- Dr. Ralph Moss
- Ulrich Abel and chemotherapy
- Chemotherapy for breast cancer
- Risks of chemotherapy for breast cancer
- Complications from chemotherapy for breast cancer
- Does chemotherapy affect overall survival for breast cancer?
- Dr. Susan Love and chemotherapy
- Does chemotherapy cure breast cancer?

As I've mentioned earlier, Dr. Russell Blaylock's books are good reference. His book, *Natural Strategies for Cancer Patients*, will show you how to minimize some of the side effects of chemotherapy and how to make your treatments more effective.

We will be ready to seek a new way if we recognize that doctors can only know so much, that medicine is not an accumulation of absolute truths.

ELLEN J. LANGER, AUTHOR OF *COUNTER CLOCKWISE*

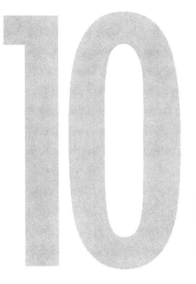

Radiation: The Nuclear War on Cancer

At least 50 percent of all women diagnosed with breast cancer, including those with diagnoses of DCIS, a pre-cancerous condition, undergo radiation therapy. Seventy-three percent of the women I surveyed had radiation therapy.

When I was diagnosed, my doctor concluded I was most likely at low risk of recurrence, but in case I was at moderate or high risk for recurrence and because of my unusual pathology and my concerns over radiation, he wanted me to meet with a radiation oncologist. So I did.

The radiation oncologist agreed with the need for the lumpectomy to determine my risk, ordered an MRI, and tried to convince me of the benefits of radiation, if it turned out that my risk for recurrence was moderate or high. After leaving his office I decided that maybe I should really reconsider the radiation; maybe these doctors did know best. So, I set out to do even more research on radiation. What I found was that my doctors had not really presented me with a full picture.

Radiation can kill cells. It can also cause cancer; the American Cancer Society lists it as a known carcinogen. The key question is: Can radiation kill cancer cells without causing cancer? The answer is: Sometimes, but not always.

Because of studies of the survivors of the atomic bombings in Japan, we know for certain that radiation exposure causes cancer. We also know that unlike leukemia, which typically develops within five years of exposure to radiation, cancers like breast cancer can take as long as ten to twenty years to develop after exposure. How can we know whether breast cancer that recurs many years after radiation therapy is a new cancer caused by the radiation itself or a recurrence of the original cancer? We can't.

We do know that the effects of radiation exposure are cumulative; they build up over time. One radiologist I talked to said that we really don't know if even very small amounts of radiation can cause cancer only because we don't live long enough for the damage to show up. We do know that the greater the exposure, the sooner the cancer occurs. Some doctors think that even the cumulative radiation exposure from mammograms may be harmful.

Like chemotherapy, radiation cannot kill all cancer cells. In the 1930s Maurice Lenz, a US pioneer in treating cancer with radiation, used doses of 6,000-8,000 rads to treat women with breast cancer. By today's standards, these are extremely high doses. Even with these high doses, cancer cells survived in the breast tissue. So, we know that the lower doses used today cannot kill all cancer cells. Oxygen is also necessary for radiation to kill cells. Because cancer cells in breast milk ducts (like DCIS) have little oxygen, they are resistant to radiation. Studies being done in which doctors increase a woman's oxygen levels during radiation treatments have been shown to make the treatments more effective.

While radiation therapy is not a systemic therapy like chemotherapy, radiation therapy still damages healthy cells. The newer radiation therapies are more targeted and concentrated on the tumor, but they cannot selectively target only the cancer cells as women are often led to believe. Normal, healthy cells within the radiation field will also be damaged. This may also include damage to cells in the heart and lungs. And some cancer cells will survive.

Any damage to healthy cells increases the risk of those cells later becoming cancer cells. So, radiation therapy has some serious long-term and short-term risks.

Because of the damage caused to healthy cells, mammograms after radiation are harder to read, making recurrences more difficult to detect. This difficulty in reading the mammograms may be one reason why a recurrence is often undetected until it has become invasive. The damage to healthy cells also prevents a woman from being able to have immediate breast reconstruction should she later need to have a mastectomy.

One study, co-authored by one of the leading breast cancer doctors, Melvin J. Silverstein, found a higher incidence of invasive cancer in women who had undergone radiation therapy for DCIS. It is not known if the invasive cancer was caused by the radiation itself or if, due to the tissue damage caused by the radiation, the cancer was simply not able to be detected until it had invaded breast tissue.

Radiation therapy for cancer is called ionizing radiation. It works in two ways: either by fatally damaging the DNA of the cell and causing almost instant death, or by creating free radicals that damage the cells over time and hopefully lead to cell death or the inability to reproduce. However, if these free radicals don't cause cell death, they can instead cause just enough damage to create a new cancer cell.

A Cornell University study of general radiation exposure concludes that radiation exposure does increase a woman's risk of breast cancer, especially for women exposed prior to menopause. While this report felt the risk of radiation-induced breast cancer was about equal to or less than other risk factors, it did acknowledge an increased risk for women under age forty-five receiving radiation therapy. According to the report, "It is accepted that radiation exposure of premenopausal women does increase the risk of developing a new breast cancer in the future, but this risk should be balanced or placed in perspective with the survival benefit from receiving the treatment."

There is a growing debate in the medical community about when radiation should be recommended, especially when the diagnosis is DCIS. Many doctors are backing away from the current standard of care that seems to schedule every woman with breast cancer for radiation therapy, regardless of her risk of recurrence. This debate started several years ago, but many oncologists still routinely order radiation for all women. A recent *New York Times* article highlights this debate. In the article

This study was published in the *American Journal of Surgery*, Volume 196, Issue 4, pages 552-555, in October 2008. The title of the article is "Invasive Local Recurrence Increased After Radiation Therapy for Ductal Carcinoma In Situ."

Here is a Web site on radiation, free radicals, and new cancer cells: http://envirocancer.cornell.edu/factsheet/physical/fs52.radiation.cfm. It includes the report published by Cornell University.

Dr. Patrick L. Borgen, chief of breast service, Department of Surgery at Memorial Sloan-Kettering Cancer Center in New York, states, "Recommending or not recommending radiation therapy has extremely significant consequences for women." He argues against radiating all women.

SIDE EFFECTS AND COMPLICATIONS

Because radiation therapy for breast cancer can cause some serious health problems, only women who will truly benefit from the treatment should consider it. What are those side effects and complications?

Side effects of Radiation Therapy
- Tissue damage to radiated breast (damage to healthy breast cells)
- Short term skin irritation
- Fatigue

Complications
- Heart damage. According to the British medical journal, *The Lancet,* radiation reduces death from breast cancer by 13.2 percent but increases death from other causes, mainly heart disease, by 21.2 percent.
- Lung disease
- Lymphedema (permanent swelling of the arm). The risk for lymphedema following breast cancer surgery doubles with radiation.

Several of the women I surveyed were still suffering from fatigue fifteen months after receiving radiation. This fatigue could be a symptom of undiagnosed heart damage. I strongly encourage any woman who is experiencing long-term fatigue after radiation to ask for tests for heart damage.

DUCTAL CARCINOMA IN SITU: THE NON-CANCER CANCER

Due to the routine use of mammography since the 1980s, previously undetectable DCIS is now commonly discovered. That might sound good—something that leads to the earlier detection of this cancer. But DCIS is not breast cancer. DCIS is a pre-cancerous condition that does not necessarily become invasive cancer. I met with three doctors before they told me this fact.

The fact that DCIS does not always progress to become invasive breast cancer was discovered through autopsies of elderly women who died from other causes. From 5 to 7.5 percent of these women had DCIS, but not invasive breast cancer. Women in Japan have incidences of DCIS slightly less than those of American women, but they have the lowest breast cancer rates in the world. American women have the highest. Although DCIS can become invasive cancer if it breaks through the wall of the milk duct, it doesn't always do that. It is not known in what percentage of women this breakthrough will occur.

Ductal carcinoma in situ (DCIS) is routinely treated with radiation. But radiation treatment for DCIS is controversial. Of all types of "breast cancer" (even though DCIS is not actually breast cancer), the least is known about DCIS and how it behaves. Therefore, personal research is especially important following a DCIS diagnosis.

As indicated in the following quotations from the introduction to the bible on DCIS, *Ductal Carcinoma in Situ of the Breast*, edited by Dr. Melvin Silverstein, doctors are in the middle of a DCIS learning curve:

- "Until 1980, DCIS was a rare disease, representing less than 1 percent of all breast cancer."
- "DCIS is not run-of-the-mill or ordinary breast cancer. Rather, it is a heterogeneous group of lesions whose diagnosis, understanding, and treatment require special knowledge and expertise."
- "Today patients with DCIS who obtain multiple consultations often get multiple different opinions regarding treatment options."

Too little time has passed since the first diagnosis of DCIS to fully understand this disease. When it was first discovered, all women with DCIS were advised to have a mastectomy. Now that practice is no longer considered appropriate. Today, all women are advised to have radiation. Now that practice, too, is being called into question.

To understand why DCIS is not considered breast cancer, read an article by Dr. Melvin Silverstein, "Ductal Carcinoma of the Breast: Controversial Issues," at http://theoncologist. alphamedpress.org/cgi/content/full/3/2/94.

You may want to consider this book for further research: *Ductal Carcinoma in Situ of The Breast* edited by Dr. Melvin J. Silverstein, medical director and senior surgical oncologist at The Breast Center in Van Nuys, California. This book contains studies on DCIS from 116 leading doctors and researchers involved with breast cancer. I used this book for much of my research when my diagnosis was just DCIS.

VAN NUYS SCALE

By using factors in your pathology report, such as the size of the DCIS, the nuclear grade, the size of clear margins, and your age, and then applying this information to the Van Nuys Scale, your doctor can determine the risk of your DCIS progressing to invasive cancer. This scale rates risk from the lowest risk (4 through 6) to the highest risk (10 through 12). Due to the potentially life-threatening complications from radiation therapy (or chemotherapy—some doctors prescribe chemotherapy for DCIS), you need to know your risk before making any decision about radiation.

Index	1	2	3
Tumor Size	0-14 mm	15-40 mm	>40 mm
Cell type and necrosis	Low and intermediate nuclear grade without necrosis	Intermediate nuclear grade with necrosis	High nuclear grade with necrosis
Extent of clear margins	>10 mm	1-9 mm	<1 mm
Age	>60	40-60	<40

To calculate your risk score on the Van Nuys Scale, take each of the four criteria listed down the left side of the scale (tumor size, cell type, margins, and your age) and find the category to the right of that criteria that matches your pathology. The score (1, 2 or 3) associated with the category you fall in is listed across the top of the scale. For example, a 6 mm tumor scores a one. You will calculate your score for each of the four criteria. Then, you add up those four scores, and that is your risk level.

Studies are showing that women determined to be at low risk for recurrence have no benefit from receiving radiation. Yet, many women whose DCIS would never have progressed to invasive cancer are receiving radiation treatments. And remember, though low, there is a risk of the radiation actually causing cancer.

On the other hand, many women who are at high risk for recurrence are simply being treated with radiation, which is not

For more information on the Van Nuys Scale, and other breast cancer topics, I recommend *The Breast Cancer Survival Manual* by John L. Link, MD.

effective for high risk DCIS when they should instead have a mastectomy. Mastectomy does offer 100 percent disease-free survival for all women with DCIS.

Dr. John R. Lee and Dr. David M. Derry are among the many doctors who think that DCIS is the result of a systemic imbalance, either estrogen dominance/progesterone deficiency and/or iodine deficiency. (Iodine deficiency can cause the hormonal imbalance.) If those imbalances can be corrected, DCIS is unlikely to progress to invasive cancer. The high iodine intake of Japanese women (who have the lowest breast cancer rate in the world) appears to be the reason their DCIS does not become invasive breast cancer. DCIS will not kill; only invasive cancer can metastasize. If you are at low or moderate risk as determined by your score on the Van Nuys Scale, taking many steps outlined in the prevention section of this book, including treating your hormonal imbalance and iodine deficiency, offers a good chance of preventing your DCIS from progressing to an invasive stage.

Your doctor may not warn you of all the risks associated with radiation treatments. If you have DCIS, they might not even calculate your risk score on the Van Nuys Scale. They didn't calculate it for me; I had to discover it through my own research. After I brought it to the attention of my doctors, they acknowledged the importance of determining my level of risk before proceeding with treatment recommendations.

When facing the option of radiation treatment, know your cancer risks, know the risks of radiation, weigh the advantages and disadvantages, and make an informed decision.

GOOGLE SEARCH SUGGESTIONS

- Adverse effects of radiation for breast cancer
- Heart damage caused by radiation for breast cancer
- Radiation induced heart disease
- Side effects of radiation for breast cancer
- Risks associated with radiation for breast cancer
- Studies on radiation and breast cancer
- Van Nuys Scale and DCIS
- When is radiation recommended for DCIS?

When all is certain, there are no choices for us. If there is no doubt, there is no choice.

ELLEN J. LANGER, AUTHOR OF *COUNTER CLOCKWISE*

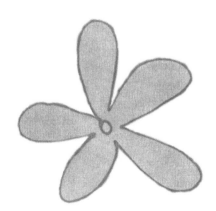

11

Mastectomy:
The Removal of Fear

Our breasts are always an issue. They are either too small or too big. As we age, they sag. They are a source of both pleasure and pain, and they are inextricably linked to our sexual identities. But, bluntly put, breasts biologically are just fat, and they are certainly not worth losing life over or even sacrificing quality of life for. While today lumpectomies followed by radiation appear to provide similar survival rates to those of mastectomies for some breast cancers, a mastectomy should still be considered along with all other treatment options. On the other hand, a mastectomy is not always the right treatment, and it may definitely be too drastic for certain diagnoses, such as low or moderate risk DCIS. However, for many breast cancer diagnoses and for nearly all cases of recurrence, it can offer the highest long-term survival rate.

Not all studies agree, however, that lumpectomy and radiation offer the same survival rates as mastectomy. In one study published in *Clinical Reviews*, 701 women were studied over twenty years; 349 women had mastectomies and 352 women had lumpectomies plus radiation. In the mastectomy group, eight women had a local recurrence (2.3 percent). In the lumpectomy group, thirty women had a local recurrence (8.8 percent).

This study was published in the January 2003 issue of *Clinical Reviews*, titled, "Studies Compare Mastectomy, Lumpectomy Survival Rates." The study is available at http://goliath. ecnext.com/coms2/gi_0199 -2605025/Studies-compare -mastectomy-lumpectomy -survival.html.

For fear of losing their breasts, many women may opt for radiation or chemotherapy when a mastectomy is warranted. This fear of a mastectomy is sometimes rooted in memories of an aunt or grandmother who had a mastectomy thirty or forty years ago. One of my employees, who is over age sixty, secretly pulled my husband aside and told him that she thought I was in denial about how bad my mastectomy surgery and recovery were actually going to be. After seeing how quickly I recovered, she confessed to me that she was basing her fear on watching her aunt recover from a radical mastectomy nearly thirty years ago. Times have changed. From the first radical mastectomies pioneered by William Stewart Halsted in the late 1880s when the theory was that more was better and women were left with large open chest wounds that took months to heal (he also suggested removal of the arm and hip in cases of metastases!), a mastectomy today is a much less invasive procedure.

Even though I knew that the surgery had changed, I was prepared for months of painful recovery—not being able to work or do my yoga practice. I prepared meals in advance and stashed them in the freezer thinking I would be unable to cook for several weeks. I was prepared for pain and Frankenstein-like scars across my chest. I had a stack of books all picked out to read during my recovery time. And I was sure I would have plenty of time to write this book while I recovered.

I expected my chest to be totally bandaged up, but when I looked down for the first time after the surgery, I had just two small gauze bandages taped across the center of my breasts. Because I opted for immediate reconstruction, I even had small "breasts"—it was almost as if I hadn't had the surgery at all. And the Frankenstein scars I had worried about were nothing more than a thin line.

I had my surgery on Friday afternoon and came home on Sunday morning. I never needed a pain pill once I left the hospital, not even an Advil. Yes, the drainage tubes were a nuisance, but they were taken out after four days. I felt guilty when friends came to visit bearing plates of food. I wasn't lying around "recovering" as we all had thought I would be. I did follow my doctor's instructions to not lift more than ten pounds and not move my arms over my head for two weeks, so there were some things that I could not do. But for the most part, after just a week I was back

:o doing 80 percent of what I did prior to surgery. Within six weeks I was back to 100 percent, even doing my full yoga practice, a strenuous routine.

I realize that not every woman's experience with mastectomy will be as easy as mine. I did ask my surgeons what the typical recovery was, and they said that recovery is generally quite fast, except for women who experience emotional distress over the loss of their breasts. These women, they said, have a much harder recovery. I have gone into a few chat rooms where women discuss their recovery, and I have discovered the experience varies some, but not a great deal. From those chat rooms I discovered that the women who suffered complications, such as infections or fluid buildup (called seroma) had not had drainage tubes inserted during surgery and/or were not prescribed an antibiotic.

MASTECTOMY DEFINED

A mastectomy is the surgical removal of the entire breast. There are four general types of mastectomy:

- Radical Mastectomy: removal of the entire breast, chest wall muscles, and lymph nodes (rarely done today)
- Modified Radical Mastectomy: removal of the breast and lymph nodes
- Simple Mastectomy: removal of the breast but not the lymph nodes
- Subcutaneous (Skin Sparing) Mastectomy: the breast is removed but the nipple and areola remain in place.

LUMPECTOMY VS. MASTECTOMY

A lumpectomy, sometimes referred to as a partial mastectomy, is the removal of breast tissue surrounding a malignant tumor or area of DCIS. Enough breast tissue is removed in order to establish an area that is free of cancer cells. This area is called the margins. (If your cancer was like an egg, the cancer would be the yolk and the margins would be the whites.) The magic number for clear margins is 10 mm. The size of your margins will appear in your pathology report. If your doctor tells you your margins were clear, be sure to ask the exact size of those margins in all directions. Anything less than 10 mm clear in all directions is considered inadequate to establish local control. Local control means treatment by removing the cancer and surrounding tissue. In all studies where lumpectomy and mastectomy were shown to offer comparable survival rates, that was only true in cases when lumpectomy was followed by radiation and only in the instance of the initial diagnosis, not following a recurrence.

To many women, a lumpectomy would seem to offer a better cosmetic result than mastectomy. I found this not to be true. In fact, I felt (and looked) more deformed after my lumpectomy than after my mastectomy. An adequate lumpectomy removes quite a bit of tissue; in some women this may leave the breast smaller or with a pronounced indentation.

When is a mastectomy recommended over lumpectomy and radiation? Mastectomy is recommended in the following instances:

- The breast cancer tumor is larger than 5 cm (50 mm).
- Two or more areas of breast cancer are far apart in the same breast, making local control via lumpectomy undesirable.
- A woman has already had radiation.
- A woman does not want to receive radiation treatments.
- Surgeons cannot establish 10 mm of clear margins through lumpectomy.
- Breast cancer tumors are large in relation to size of the breast.
- Breast cancer is a recurrence after lumpectomy.
- "Breast cancer" is multi-focal moderate-to-high-risk DCIS.

MASTECTOMY AFTER RECURRENCE

In the event of local recurrence (recurrence in the same breast) after a lumpectomy and radiation, a mastectomy clearly offers a greater survival benefit. The women who had a mastectomy following recurrence had nearly a 20 percent better survival rate than those who had a second lumpectomy.

RISKS AND COMPLICATIONS FROM MASTECTOMY

The risks associated with a mastectomy are the same as those related to any surgical procedure done under general anes-

On the Web site for breastcancer.org, you can read a review of a study published in the *American Journal of Surgery* in 2008, "The Survival Impact of the Choice of Surgical Procedure After Ipsilateral Breast Cancer Recurrence." The review of this article states "mastectomy clearly provides the maximal risk reduction in the recurrence of breast cancer because it leaves the least amount of breast tissue behind."

thesia. Unlike radiation and chemotherapy, there is no increased cancer risk or risk of damage to other organs.

Complications from mastectomy include:

- Infection (more common in the case of immediate reconstruction and when post-operative antibiotics are not prescribed)
- Fluid buildup called seroma (if drains are not inserted)
- Lymphedema (if lymph nodes are removed). A new study has just come out showing that weight lifting can reduce the incidence and/or severity of lymphedema.

Lymphedema (swelling of the arm) is the most serious of these, but none are life-threatening.

RECONSTRUCTION

Not all women who undergo mastectomy are concerned about reconstruction. But for many, the ability to have immediate reconstruction makes the decision to have a mastectomy bearable. It can also be extremely important for women who have a strong psychological attachment to their breasts; reconstruction can help with the healing process. Immediate reconstruction was certainly helpful for me.

Many women just want to deal with the mastectomy and then worry about the decision to have reconstruction or not later. However, if you are a candidate for immediate reconstruction, I would advise you to research this option and consult with a plastic surgeon experienced in breast reconstruction before your mastectomy surgery. Immediate breast reconstruction avoids a second major surgery later, and it offers better cosmetic results.

You are a candidate for immediate reconstruction if you have not had radiation therapy, are not a smoker, and have no other health complications. If you will be having chemotherapy treatments after your mastectomy, some doctors recommend delaying the reconstruction.

TYPES OF BREAST RECONSTRUCTION

Two basic types of breast reconstruction are available following a mastectomy: tissue expander and tissue transfer (called TRAM).

For reconstruction using a tissue expander, a deflated implant is inserted under the pectoral muscle at the time of the mastectomy. After you have healed from the mastectomy (usually in about three weeks), you will receive a weekly series of saline injections into the implant, which will gradually allow your skin and muscle to expand along with the implant. These injections are painless, and the result is a mild tightness in the chest while the muscle adjusts. The number of saline injections is determined by the cup size you ultimately wish to achieve. Once your body has adjusted to the size of the expander implants (this will be about three months after your last saline injection), they will be removed during a simple outpatient surgery, and the permanent implants inserted. Several months later, you can choose to have another surgery in which nipples are created, or you can simply have nipples tattooed, which is how the aerola is recreated. Although this method is called immediate reconstruction, this entire process will take from six to eighteen months.

A new version of immediate reconstruction called "skin sparing" mastectomy is also an option. This procedure removes the breast glandular tissue and nipple, but leaves a majority of the skin to envelope the implant. Because more breast tissue remains, there is a slightly higher risk of recurrence with this procedure. My surgeon mentioned this procedure to me, but as he said, if you are having a mastectomy to remove as much risk as possible of a recurrence, why take the chance with this procedure? I agreed. I had a simple mastectomy with the expander reconstruction mentioned above.

The second type of reconstruction, using the tissue transfer technique, involves relocating tissue from one area of your body to form a new breast. This procedure involves two major incisions: one in your breast and the other at the site where the other tissue is being removed. Tissue is usually taken from the back or the stomach. There are two methods of transferring this tissue. One involves "tunneling" it under the skin to the breast area, and the other, called "free transfer," allows the tissue to be completely removed and relocated to the breast area. Either method requires much more time in surgery and a much longer recovery time. Because you are moving tissue, not an implant, into the area where there were breast cancer cells, this option may also pose a higher risk of recurrence. My surgeon said that since this is a newer procedure, it is not known yet if that would be the case.

Mastectomy is clearly the appropriate treatment for some women, but it is certainly not warranted in all cases of breast cancer. Like chemotherapy and radiation, it cannot entirely remove the risk of recurrence, except in the case of DCIS. But, there are reasons to consider a mastectomy over other forms of treatment. Many women choose a mastectomy to have more peace of mind. Some choose a mastectomy because they do not want to undergo chemotherapy or radiation. And some women, with a family history of breast cancer, undergo a mastectomy as a means of prevention. As with all breast cancer treatments, it is ultimately a personal decision.

I chose to have a mastectomy because, although initially diagnosed with DCIS, invasive breast cancer and more DCIS were discovered through a lumpectomy. My lumpectomy did not obtain clear margins around either the invasive tumor or the DCIS. My breast cancer was triple negative, so would not respond to Tamoxifen. I ranked high on the Van Nuys scale—meaning my cancer was aggressive. The cancer had not spread to my lymph nodes, and I did not want it to. From all of my research I felt that radiation or chemotherapy would only do more harm and not rid me of the cancer. Because of my research, I knew that a mastectomy was the right treatment for me.

GOOGLE SEARCH SUGGESTIONS

- Mastectomy and breast reconstruction
- Types of mastectomy
- Mastectomy photos
- Breast reconstruction after mastectomy
- Types of breast reconstruction
- Risks of breast reconstruction
- Comparing lumpectomy to mastectomy
- When is a mastectomy recommended for breast cancer?
- Mastectomy after recurrence of breast cancer
- Risks associated with mastectomy
- Complications after mastectomy
- Mastectomy for genetic breast cancer

For more information on mastectomy and breast reconstruction, here are a few books that may be helpful:

Dr. Susan Love's Breast Book, 4th edition, by Susan Love, MD

Keep Your Breasts: Survive Breast Cancer by Susan H. Moss

The Breast Cancer Survival Manual by John Link, MD

The only real mistake is the one from which we learn nothing.

JOHN POWELL

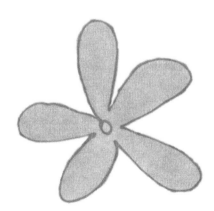

12

Breast Cancer Prevention Action Plan

On the following page, check all the statements that have applied to you over the past five to seven years—because most breast cancers take at least five years to grow to a size that is detectable. The more you check, the higher your risk. Once you have identified the areas that put you at higher risk, you can take action to remove those risks by changing those things you have the power to change. No matter what treatment you decide on, if you don't change what contributed to your breast cancer in the first place, you are much more likely to have a recurrence.

MY PERSONAL RISK FACTORS FOR BREAST CANCER

____Chronic inflammation (arthritis, allergies, yeast infections, gum disease, etc.).

____High sugar consumption (all sugars, white breads, white pastas, crackers, fruit juices, cookies, granola bars, sodas, etc.).

____Red meat consumption more than once a day.

____Low fruit and vegetable consumption.

____Low fiber consumption.

____Do not take vitamin and mineral supplements.

____Get little exercise.

____Do not eat organic produce.

____Drink milk and dairy with rBGH (most milk and dairy has rBGH unless labeled otherwise).

____Eat processed/packaged food often.

____Eat out several times a week or more.

____Low iodine consumption.

____Have symptoms of hormonal imbalances.

____Taking synthetic Hormone Replacement Therapy (HRT).

____High stress.

____Lack of sleep.

____Toxins in cosmetics.

____Family history of breast cancer.

____Overweight.

____Started menstruation early (before age 15).

____Used birth control pills for more than 15 years.

____Did not have children.

____Did not breast feed.

____Fibrocystic breasts.

____Physical injury to breast(s).

MY PERSONAL ACTION PLAN FOR REDUCING MY RISK

List the steps in your action plan in order of priority.

1. _____

2. _____

3. _____

4. _____

5. _____

6. _____

7. _____

8. _____

9. _____

10. _____

11. _____

12. _____

13. _____

14. _____

15. _____

16. _____

17. _____

18. _____

19. _____

20. _____

Begin implementing your action plan, one step at a time.

All truth passes through three stages. First, it is ridiculed. Second, it is violently opposed. Third, it is accepted as self-evident.

ARTHUR SCHOPENHAUER

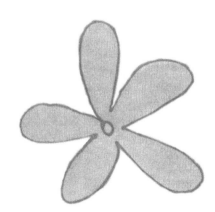

13 Postscript

There is only one constant in life: change. We witness it daily in the change of weather and seasons, in world events, and in our bodies as we age over time. Although change surrounds us, choosing to change our beliefs, our lifestyle, our diet, or the way we view doctors or the field of medicine is not easy. For some it may prove impossible.

We are attached to our beliefs, so it takes a mountain of evidence to change our belief in something. We often deny knowledge because if we accept it, we would have to change. It is easier to stay with the status quo, even if it is not working. But change is essential for growth, healing, and an expansion of knowledge.

Illness is a change thrust upon us—an unwelcome one. It is our body's way of telling us of a need for change. That's what breast cancer told me. It's what my uterine fibroid tumors were trying to tell me. When I developed fibroid tumors years ago, my body told me I needed to change, but I didn't listen until it was too late. I should have tried to find out what caused them, not just how to get rid of the symptoms. But I didn't understand the need to do my own research then. I never knew how important it was to take charge of my own health.

Then I developed breast cancer, along with a voracious hunger to understand how to survive it and prevent recurrence.

I learned that breast cancer doesn't just happen, but that something causes it. Once I knew and understood, it was easier to change.

I now know that my stressful 24/7 schedule and my iodine deficiency weakened my immune system and wreaked havoc with my hormone levels. Both the stress and the hormone imbalances contributed to my breast cancer. I needed to change my lifestyle if I did not want a recurrence. I no longer work seven days a week, and I am trying to incorporate a meditation practice into my day. I had already taken the difficult steps to change my diet several years ago. I am now working with a qualified health practitioner to re-balance my hormones and am taking iodine supplements along with a full range of other beneficial supplements I discussed in this book. I am also fully convinced of the benefits of blenderizing vegetables, and I drink them daily.

Knowledge is never complete. Research continues, and more information about breast cancer prevention and survival becomes available almost daily.

More research needs to be done and more information needs to be made available on breast cancer prevention. In my research for this book I came across many breast cancer organizations, many trying to do their part to combat this disease. One organization of note is the Dr. Susan Love Research Foundation. Dr. Susan Love is the author of several books on breast cancer and director of the UCLA Breast Center. I like her philosophy. She says, "Research is the only way we are going to solve this thing, and I don't mean research into new chemo formulas; I mean research into the cause of breast cancer."

It now appears that 90 percent of all breast cancer is preventable. With that understanding, I know you will find it easier to make the changes that will prevent you from getting breast cancer or, if already diagnosed, from having a recurrence. I also hope you found the information in this book so valuable that you will share it with all your friends, daughters, mothers, and sisters. Most of all I hope I have spurred you on to do your own research and take charge of your own health and health care decisions.

I hope you are empowered!

Sheryl Ellinwood

You can volunteer to be part of any of the research studies on breast cancer by becoming one of Dr. Love's "ARMY OF WOMEN." Go to www.dslrf.org for more information. To "meet" Dr. Susan Love, Google: *New York Times* A Day With Doctor Susan Love.

It is important to me that readers know that my personal research on breast cancer has no economic bias. I have received no compensation in any form from any source or supplier cited in this book.

Profits from the sale of this book will be used to update and maintain the Web site www.pinkempower.com. The Web site, like this book, was created in order to connect women with information on breast cancer prevention and treatments. As I discover new information and resources, I will post them on the Web site. If you have information you would like to share, you can email me through the Web site.

For easier access to the Web sites listed in this book, links to each of these URLs are available at www.pinkempower.com. In addition, information on how to purchase the PINKemPOWER Breast Cancer Bracelet and additional copies of this book is also available at this same Web site.

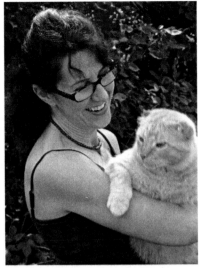

Sheryl Ellinwood with Goober,
one of her adopted stray cats.

Meet the Author

Sheryl is that rare combination of artist and businesswoman. She spent twelve years working in the health insurance field before deciding to change careers. She earned her BFA degree from the University of Toledo (Ohio) in 1991 and her MFA degree from the University of Southern Illinois (Carbondale) in 1994. She was awarded a graduate fellowship in 1993.

In 1994 she founded her business, ellinwood studios, inc. That business began with glassblowing and evolved into the creation of jewelry and home décor that is sold in shops and galleries across the country. Another aspect of Sheryl's business is creating large commissioned glass wall pieces for major adult and children's hospitals.

Sheryl's personal artistic work takes the form of mixed-media sculptures influenced by science, philosophy, nature, and various religious belief systems. Her sculptures are in many galleries and in corporate, public, and private collections. She is both an avid reader and traveler. Her most recent travels include trips to South Africa, Thailand, Laos, Cambodia, and Vietnam.

Sheryl's research into cancer and its treatments and prevention began more than a year before she was diagnosed with breast cancer. When someone close to her was diagnosed with melanoma, she immediately began researching the disease and less toxic, more effective treatments than those offered under the current standard of care. When she herself was diagnosed with cancer, she continued her research, focusing on breast cancer.

Sheryl's breast cancer diagnosis inspired her not only to write this book, but also to create a breast cancer bracelet, the Pink emPOWER bracelet (bracelet information available at www.pinkempower.com).

Sheryl practices yoga and is passionate about health, good food, and cooking. Sheryl and her husband, Jerome (Jerry) Keller, live and work together in rural Iowa. Together they tend a large, organic garden. They presently have three cats, Smooch, Goober, and Cancer Kitty, all rescued strays.

For more information on ellinwood studios, visit www.ellinwoodstudios.com.

For more information about the Pink emPOWER project, visit www.pinkempower.com.

Index

A

ACS 22, 31, 85, 87
adjuvant chemotherapy 23
adrenal glands 70, 71
agave nectar 41
Akt 38
allergies 43, 58, 128
allopathic 31, 32, 36, 76
alternative medicine 32, 76
AMA 86
American Cancer Society 9, 76, 63, 83, 87,
        89, 87, 111
American Medical Association 20, 63, 85, 86
antidepressants 63, 38, 59
anti-inflammatory 49
apoptosis 29
AstraZeneca 84, 88

B

banned 44, 48, 61, 62, 87
berries 46
BHRT 78, 80
bioidentical hormones 72, 73, 74, 75, 77, 80
biopsy 27, 93
birth control pills 72, 128
blenderize vegetables 46
Breast Cancer Awareness Month 88
breast feeding 60

C

cancer cells 20, 21, 23, 27, 29, 31, 32, 36, 38,
        43, 46, 49, 55, 57, 58, 59, 76, 91, 105,
        106, 108, 111, 112, 113, 121, 124
carbohydrates 39, 51, 79
carcinogen 30, 66, 111
carcinogens 31, 61
catechins 50, 20
cells 11, 21, 36, 37, 38, 39, 43, 46, 49, 55, 56,
        57, 58, 59, 60, 70, 71, 76, 80, 91, 100,
        105, 106, 108, 111, 112, 113, 114, 113,
        121, 124
chemotherapy 18, 50, 36, 50, 49, 56, 57, 85,
        92, 93, 98, 99, 100, 101, 102, 103, 104,
        105, 106, 107, 108, 109, 112, 116, 120,
        123, 125
complications 101, 102, 105, 106, 114, 116,
        121, 123
consensus 95
continuing education 86, 49
cooking 43, 64, 71, 66, 135
corrupt 84
cortisol 64, 58, 66
cosmetics 37, 128
cumulative 112
curcumin 50

D

dairy 35, 43, 44, 45, 44, 45, 48, 44, 128
DCIS 19, 20, 26, 27, 60, 93, 102, 111, 112,
        113, 114, 115, 116, 117, 115, 119, 121,
        122, 125
DDT 48, 88
DHEA 70, 29, 71, 80
differentiated 29, 71, 24
digestive enzymes 58
diosgenin 74, 63
DNA damage 37, 74
drug companies 22, 73, 83, 84, 85, 86, 88, 89,
        91, 104
Ductal Carcinoma in Situ 114, 115

E

endocrine 61, 107
enzymes 31, 24, 58, 59
epidemic 24
epidemiology 24, 44
ER 38, 107
estradiol 70, 37, 78, 108
estriol 70, 78
estrogen 19, 78, 69, 70, 72, 79, 103, 107, 108,
        117
estrone 70, 65
exercise 64, 78, 128
expander 123, 124

F

fatigue 106, 114
fats 35, 38, 39, 84, 85, 87, 89, 88
FDA 13, 61, 64, 71, 46, 39, 46, 59, 101, 104
fear 96, 120
fiber 39, 13, 39, 46, 66, 71, 79, 128
fibrocystic breasts 60, 66, 71
fibroid tumors 40, 39, 40, 71, 47, 49, 40, 131
flavonoids 31, 40, 45, 46, 38
food 25, 45, 35, 37, 72, 86, 120, 128, 135
Food and Drug Administration 6, 30, 32, 64, 71, 46
food storage 51, 24
fraud 84
free radicals 37, 53, 45, 113
fruits 39, 37
funding 13, 45

G

glycemic index 40, 41
grains 39, 43
green tea 49, 50

H

hair dyes 87
heart damage 106, 107, 114
HER-2 19, 23
HER2-negative 21, 23
HER-2/neu 19, 59
HER2-positive 108
herbs 33, 14
homeopathy 75, 40, 32, 37, 76, 40, 44, 45, 48, 62
hormone balance 14, 77
hormone imbalance 14, 40, 73, 74
hormone receptor 20, 72
hormones 14, 78, 132
hormone test 61
HRT 71, 128

I

IJC 87
immune system 23, 66, 91, 103, 104, 105, 108, 132
implants 43, 64, 124
infection 30, 24
inflammation 43, 20, 43, 50, 58, 128
inflammatory 42, 43, 49

influence 24, 43, 84, 85, 86, 89
insulin 39, 21, 39
insulin resistance 39, 40, 41
invasive 18, 39, 93, 113, 115, 116, 117, 120, 125
in vitro 21
in vivo 21, 59
iodine 59, 61, 117, 128, 132
iodine test 61, 57
ionizing radiation 113
iron 57

J

Japanese women 60, 117

K

kickbacks 85, 86, 89
killer cells 30, 71

L

labels 40, 41, 43, 51, 52, 53, 61, 72
lawsuit 18, 95
leukemia 106, 107, 112
liability 6, 96
local control 121, 122
lumpectomy 12, 20, 119, 121, 122, 125, 120
lymphedema 114, 123
lymph nodes 27, 121, 123, 125

M

mammogram 12, 20, 26, 65, 66, 79
margins 27, 116, 121, 122, 125, 121, 122, 125
marketing 63, 84, 86, 89
mastectomy 79
meat 35, 20, 24, 44, 128
medical studies 11, 27, 20, 27
melatonin 65
metastasis 59, 103
misleading 51, 101, 102, 104
Modified citrus pectin 59
MRI 20, 111

N

nail polish 62
nanobees 76
nanotechnology 76
National Cancer Institute 9, 23, 50, 83, 87, 89, 106

NCI 22, 49, 85, 87
necrosis 116
NF-Kappa B 49
non-toxic 13
nuclear grade 116

O

oils 43
omega-3 43
omega-6 42, 43
oncologist 23, 92, 93, 102, 103, 106, 108, 109, 111, 115
organic 44, 45, 46, 48, 53, 52, 60, 128, 135
oxidation 37, 38
oxygen 38, 65, 112

P

patentable 25, 50
pathology 8, 11, 17, 19, 20, 26, 27, 29, 92, 93, 94, 111, 116, 121
pattern recognition 92, 93
peer pressure 95
perimenopausal 64
pesticides 37, 21
petro-chemicals 42
PET scan 38
Pfizer 84, 61, 51
pharma 84, 32
phytoestrogens 44
pink ribbon 31, 36
placebo 21, 72
plastics 37, 64
PR 44
pre-cancerous 20, 93, 111, 114
Prempro 63, 38, 75, 51
prescription drugs 31, 71, 84
prevention 9, 38, 74, 108, 117, 125, 132, 133, 135
profits 32
progesterone 19, 117
protein 19, 108

R

radiation 18, 19, 22, 26, 27, 31, 32, 33, 36, 39, 56, 57, 66, 57, 77, 93, 95, 105, 106, 107, 111, 112, 113, 114, 115, 116, 117, 113, 114, 119, 120, 122, 123, 125
radiation exposure 112, 113

randomized 21, 22, 24
receptor 19, 20, 38, 63, 77, 103
reconstruction 43, 113, 120, 123, 124, 125
recurrence 9, 26, 31, 35, 36, 35, 36, 55, 57, 55, 57, 93, 111, 112, 113, 116, 111, 112, 113, 116, 125, 119, 122, 124, 125, , 122, 119, 122, 124, 125, 124, 122, 127, 131, 132, 131, 132
representativeness errors 94
Resveratrol 49, 50
risk factors 40, 113

S

saliva test 73, 74, 79
seaweed 60
second opinion 75, 109
side effects 18, 39, 101, 102, 105, 106, 108, 109, 114
simple sugars 38, 39, 46
SLAPP 45, 53
sleep 64, 65, 71, 128
soda 42, 31
soy 44, 49
spices 46, 49, 74, 37
statistics 14, 27, 102, 104, 106
stevia 41, 64, 65
stress 64, 38, 69, 71, 78, 128, 132
sugar 35, 36, 55, 56, 57, 58, 59, 57, 78, 71, 78, 128
sulforaphane 58
supplements 32, 27, 74, 75, 96, 128, 132
survival 13, 102, 103, 107, 109, 113, 117, 119, 122, 120, 132
survival rate 102, 119, 122
systemic 112, 117

T

Tamoxifen 12, 14, 44, 79, 107, 108, 125
Taxanes 106
Taxol 21, 8, 23, 106, 107
T cells 30
testing 61, 71, 37
testosterone 70, 71
thyroid hormone 59, 37
tissue damage 27, 113
tissue transfer 123, 124
toxins 31
treatments 8, 102, 108, 122, 123, 125, 133, 135

triple negative 94, 116, 125
tumor size 101

U

uncertainty 95
undifferentiated 29

V

Van Nuys Scale 116, 117, 116
vegetables 39, 40, 43, 45, 46, 56, 64, 80, 132
vitamins 45, 55, 56

W

Wall Street 87
water 25, 65, 71
weight 64, 71, 51, 123
weight gain 64, 40
whole wheat 40

X

xenoestrogens 37, 38, 48, 50, 61, 62, 70

Y

yam 74

LaVergne, TN USA
30 September 2009

159437LV00003B/2/P